Studies in language disability and remediation 6

General editors:

David Crystal
Professor of Linguistic Science, University of Reading

Jean Cooper
Principal of the National Hospitals College of Speech Sciences, London

Also published in this series:

1 The grammatical analysis of language disability:
a procedure for assessment and remediation

David Crystal, Paul Fletcher and Michael Garman

1A Working with LARSP

David Crystal

2 Phonological disability in children

David Ingram

3 Disorders of fluency and their effects on communication

Peggy Dalton and W.J. Hardcastle

4 Linguistic investigations of aphasia

Ruth Lesser

5 Language and disadvantage

John R. Edwards

Aphasia Therapy

Edited by Chris Code and Dave J. Müller

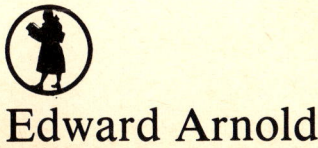

Edward Arnold

©Edward Arnold (Publishers) Ltd 1983

First published 1983 by Edward Arnold (Publishers) Ltd
41 Bedford Square, London WC1B 3DQ

British Library Cataloguing in Publication Data

Code, Chris
   Aphasia therapy.—(Studies in language disability
and remediation. ISSN 0144-3127; 6)
   1. Aphasia
   I. Title   II. Müller, D.J.   III. Series
   616.85′5206   RC425

ISBN 0-7131-6369-0

RC
425
.A67
1983

All rights reserved. No part of this publication may be reproduced, stored in a retrieval system, or transmitted in any form or by any means, electronic, mechanical, photo-copying, recording or otherwise, without the prior permission of Edward Arnold (Publishers) Ltd.

Text set in 10/12 pt Times Compugraphic by Colset Private Ltd, Singapore.
Printed and bound in Great Britain by Richard Clay (The Chaucer Press) Limited, Bungay, Suffolk.

Contents

	List of Contributors	vii
	General Preface	ix
	Preface	1
1	**Perspectives in Aphasia Therapy: An Overview** *Chris Code and Dave J. Müller*	2
	The Efficacy of Aphasia Therapy	14
2	Researching into the Efficacy of Aphasia Therapy *Rachel M. David*	15
	Neuropsychological Perspectives	25
3	Therapeutic Implications of Neuropsychology *Harry W. Purser*	26
4	Hemispheric Specialization Retraining: Possibilities and Problems *Chris Code*	42
	Linguistic Perspectives	60
5	Some Applications of Linguistics to Aphasia Therapy *Frances M. Hatfield and Christina Shewell*	61
6	Facilitation of Word Retrieval in Aphasia *Karalyn Patterson, Christina Purell and John Morton*	76
	Psychosocial Perspectives	88
7	An Application of Psychotherapeutic Techniques to the Management of Aphasia *Shelagh Brumfitt and Peter Clarke*	89
8	Interpersonal Perceptions of Psychosocial Adjustment to Aphasia *Dave J. Müller and Chris Code*	101
9	Group Therapy: A Learning Situation *Margaret Fawcus*	113
10	The Use of Volunteers in the Treatment of Dysphasia Following Cerebro-Vascular Accident *Margaret S. Meikle and Enid Wechsler*	120

Specific Approaches for Specific Problems 127
11 Treatment of Articulatory Apraxia in Aphasic Patients
   Susan Huskins 128
12 Acoustic Analysis and Auditory Retraining in the Remediation of Sensory Aphasia
   Elizabeth J. Gielewski 138
13 The Treatment of Pure Alexia
   Rowena Godwin 146
14 Aspects of Acquired Dysgraphia and Implications for Re-education
   Frances M. Hatfield 157

Alternative Communication Methods 170
15 Artificial Languages and Communication Aids in Aphasia Therapy
   David T. Rowley 171
16 Blissymbolics and Aphasia Therapy: A Case Study
   Stella Bailey 178
17 Communication Aid and Therapeutic Tool: A Report on the Clinical Trial Using Splink with Aphasic Patients
   Pam Enderby and Guy Hamilton 187

18 **Aphasia Therapy Research: A Single-Case Study Approach** 193
   Max Coltheart

References 203
Subject Index 221
Author Index 225

Contributors

Stella Bailey
Chief Speech Therapist, Torbay Health Authority, Devon
Shelagh Brumfitt
Lecturer in Language Pathology, University of Sheffield
Peter Clarke
Senior Lecturer in Clinical Psychology, University of Sheffield
Chris Code
Lecturer in Speech Pathology and Neurolinguistics, Leicester Polytechnic
Max Coltheart
Professor of Psychology, Birkbeck College, London
Rachel David
Lecturer in Speech Pathology, Central School of Speech and Drama, London
Pam Enderby
Chief Speech Therapist, Frenchay Hospital, Bristol
Margaret Fawcus
Senior Lecturer, Centre for Clinical Communication Disorders, London
Elizabeth Gielewski
Senior Speech Therapist, Royal Talbot General Rehabilitation Hospital, Victoria, Australia
Rowena Godwin
Lecturer in Speech Pathology, City of Manchester College of Higher Education
Guy Hamilton
General Practitioner, Woking
Frances M. Hatfield
Senior Speech Therapist, Addenbrooke's Hospital, Cambridge
Susan Huskins
Lecturer in Speech Pathology, Birmingham Polytechnic
Margaret S. Meikle
Chief Speech Therapist, Northwick Park Hospital, Harrow
John Morton
MRC Applied Psychology Unit, Cambridge
Dave J. Müller
Senior Lecturer in Psychology, South Glamorgan Institute of Higher Education, Cardiff

Karalyn Patterson
  MRC Applied Psychology Unit, Cambridge
Christina Purell
  Research Speech Therapist, MRC Applied Psychology Unit, Cambridge
Harry W. Purser
  Senior Lecturer in Psychology, Leicester Polytechnic
David T. Rowley
  Lecturer in Psychology, Leicester Polytechnic
Christina Shewell
  Senior Speech Therapist, Addenbrooke's Hospital, Cambridge
Enid Wechsler
  Chief Speech Therapist, University College Hospital, London

General Preface

This series is the first to approach the problem of language disability as a single field. It attempts to bring together areas of study which have traditionally been treated under separate headings, and to focus on the common problems of analysis, assessment and treatment which characterize them. Its scope therefore includes the specifically linguistic aspects of the work of such areas as speech therapy, remedial teaching, teaching of the deaf and educational psychology, as well as those aspects of mother-tongue and foreign-language teaching which pose similar problems. The research findings and practical techniques from each of these fields can inform the others, and we hope one of the main functions of this series will be to put people from one profession into contact with the analogous situations found in others.

It is therefore not a series about specific syndromes or educationally narrow problems. While the orientation of a volume is naturally towards a single main area, and reflects an author's background, it is editorial policy to ask authors to consider the implications of what they say for the fields with which they have not been primarily concerned. Nor is this a series about disability in general. The medical, social, educational and other factors which enter into a comprehensive evaluation of any problems will not be studied as ends in themselves, but only in so far as they bear directly on the understanding of the nature of the language behaviour involved. The aim is to provide a much needed emphasis on the description and analysis of language as such, and on the provision of specific techniques of therapy or remediation. In this way, we hope to bridge the gap between the theoretical discussion of 'causes' and the practical tasks of treatment—two sides of language disability which it is uncommon to see systematically related.

Despite restricting the area of disability to specifically linguistic matters—and in particular emphasizing problems of the production and comprehension of spoken language—it should be clear that the series' scope goes considerably beyond this. For the first books, we have selected topics which have been particularly neglected in recent years, and which seem most able to benefit from contemporary research in linguistics and its related disciplines, English studies, psychology, sociology and education. Each volume will put its subject matter in perspective, and will provide an introductory slant to its presentation. In this way, we hope to provide specialized studies which can be used as texts for components of teaching courses, as well as material that is directly applicable to the needs of professional workers. It is also hoped that this orientation will place the series within the reach of the interested layman—in particular, the parents or family of the linguistically disabled.

David Crystal
Jean Cooper

Preface

The idea for this book grew out of a conference on aphasia therapy which was held on 19 and 20 July, 1980, at the South Glamorgan Institute of Higher Education, Cardiff. This conference, which was organized by the editors, was conceived in the first place to provide a forum for the discussion of therapeutic approaches to the problem of acquired aphasia. In the past there have been conferences and volumes devoted to aphasia, but these have usually been predominantly concerned with aspects of description and assessment, and have given only passing reference to the problems of rehabilitation. This situation is slowly changing however, with recent times seeing an increase in concern for rehabilitation.

In preparing the book the main concern has been to present a comprehensive discussion of the contemporary issues in aphasia therapy, together with constructive consideration of a number of specific therapeutic approaches to a wide range of aphasic problems. A number of chapters in the book were presented at the conference, while others are contributions which have been specially invited to achieve a balanced and comprehensive coverage. Assessment and theory are considered only in terms of their contribution to treatment. Special consideration is also given to the currently developing fields of psychosocial adjustment, psychotherapy and the applications of neuropsychological knowledge and techniques to aphasia rehabilitation and the problems of evaluating the effectiveness of therapeutic intervention. The book should therefore be of relevance and interest to therapists, researchers, lecturers and students in the fields of speech pathology/communication disorders, clinical and neuropsychology and neuro- and psycholinguistics.

The editors wish to express their gratitude to a number of individuals and organizations for help in the organization of the original conference which gave rise to this book, and for help in the preparation of the book itself. Thanks are due to Carol Miller for chairing the conference so effectively, to Ailsa Lewis, Sue Booth, Sally Penrose and Jayne Easton for acting as stewards, and to Medilec Ltd, Photographic Teaching Materials, NFER Publishing and the Chest, Heart and Stroke Association for financial sponsorship. In the preparation of the book thanks are due to Lynne Conway for help with typing, to Julia Hawkins for general help and to the Series Editors, David Crystal and Jean Cooper, and Sarah Barrett of Edward Arnold for support and guidance throughout preparation.

C.C.
D.J.M.
April, 1982.

Perspectives in Aphasia Therapy: An Overview

This introductory chapter presents an overview of aphasia therapy which attempts to bring together the contributions of the relevant disciplines, models and approaches which are represented in this volume. An emphasis is placed on the eclectic and interdisciplinary nature of aphasia therapy, drawing as it does on a number of theoretical perspectives.

1
Perspectives in aphasia therapy: an overview
Chris Code and Dave J. Müller

Introduction

The history of aphasia therapy is short. The traditional repertoire of therapeutic procedures has been developed in response to the apparent needs of patients and reflects developments and research in a number of fields. Aphasia therapy has been influenced by trends and ideas which have permeated through from the general field of human behaviour and from other applied areas of the behavioural sciences. Consequently, therapeutic approaches to aphasia are by necessity heuristic in nature, having been derived from education, linguistics, psychology and other branches of clinical speech pathology. These approaches are characterized by a number of broad perspectives, some of which are traditional and well established, whereas the contribution of others has yet to be determined.

The argument advanced here is that aphasia therapists should be aware of at least six perspectives. The first perspective is that aphasia therapy should take credence of a fully qualitative appreciation of an individual's difficulties in linguistic terms and assumes that the observable characteristics of aphasia can be described and remediated in terms of a linguistic methodology. The second perspective accepts that the complementary nonverbal aspects of communication, which are essential features of human interaction, should be fully evaluated in aphasic individuals and considered in relationship to therapy.

The third perspective acknowledges that aphasia, while an observable language disorder, is caused by brain damage, and that underlying the linguistic disturbance is a disruption of neuropsychological processing. This emphasizes that language processing is intimately related to and dependent upon the higher cortical functions of movement (praxia), perception (gnosis) and memory (mnesis). Therefore, therapy should be planned with careful consideration given to the significance of disrupted neurocognitive mechanisms for the individual patient and their possible function in rehabilitation.

The fourth perspective is an appreciation that aphasia causes more than a linguistic disorder which occurs in isolation, and produces serious psychosocial reactions which affect the patient's entire social existence. It is suggested that these psychosocial factors should no longer be considered as 'secondary' effects of aphasia but central problems which require the active attention of the aphasia therapist. Included in this is an appreciation that rehabilitation means more than clinical improvement. Progress can only be genuine if generalized to the individual's environment. Implicit in this is that therapeutic approaches based on naturalistic or semi-naturalistic situations may have a special contribution to make to this problem of generalization.

A fifth perspective is that therapy is more likely to be effective when planned and carried out in terms of a systematic behavioural hierarchy. Utilization of a behavioural methodology recognizes that the application of techniques such as reinforcement, prompting and fading are fundamental components of treatment and should be written into any therapeutic programme before treatment begins.

The sixth perspective of this eclectic approach is the need for careful ongoing evaluation of the patient's changing state along linguistic, nonverbal, neuropsychological, behavioural and psychosocial parameters in parallel with therapy. This means that treatment programmes should be under constant session-by-session review and modification in the light of both the patient's and therapist's performance. Thus it is advocated that an hypothesis-testing approach to treatment methods and materials should be adopted.

These six perspectives are assumed to be essential elements which are seen as having more or less equal status and importance in aphasia rehabilitation. It is suggested that the aphasia therapist should design a therapeutic programme based upon a linquistic, nonverbal and neuropsychological perspective of the patient's difficulties, and should present tasks within a systematic behavioural strategy, whilst bearing in mind the patient's psychosocial state and requirements. In parallel with this, the therapist should conduct an ongoing evaluation of the patient's responses and set up hypotheses for testing, which will subsequently modify treatment.

A linguistic perspective

Linguistic investigations of aphasic language have contributed much to our understanding of the nature of aphasia (see Lesser 1978, for a review) and a description of the patient's communicative abilities along linguistic parameters would appear to be essential before treatment can be planned. Such a description, as well as the treatment based upon it, need not necessarily require the therapist to accept some of the more abstract linguistic explanations of aphasic language (Jakobson 1964; 1968; Kean 1977). However, an understanding of some linguistic notions which have received much attention in neurolinguistic research may serve as a practical basis for linguistic approaches to therapy; in particular, the fundamental linguistic dichotomies of selection and combination, competence and performance, and propositional and non-propositional language.

The *selection-combination* dichotomy was first applied to aphasic language by Jakobson (1956) and represents the fundamental opposition of the *paradigmatic* (selection) and *syntagmatic* (combination) aspects of language. Jakobson (1964) also used the terms *similarity* (selection) and *contiguity* (combination).

In essence, when applied to aphasia, this dichotomy refers to a disorder at either the *paradigmatic level*, where a patient for instance, may have problems with word-finding or phonemic access (*selection*), or an impairment of the *syntagmatic level* where there are difficulties stringing together linguistic elements, such as phonemes into words or words into sentences (*combination*). Clearly, patients may have impairment at both levels, but by way of illustration, a pure anomic patient may be usefully described as having a predominantly selection disorder, and a patient with agrammatism as having a combination disorder. The therapeutic implication of relation and combination are discussed by Hatfield and Shewell (chapter 5).

Some neurolinguistic theorists consider that linguistic *competence* (a speaker's underlying tacit knowledge of the language) remains intact in aphasia (Weigl and Bierwisch 1970) and it is only linguistic *performance* (the speakers actual use of language) which is affected. Whitaker, on the other hand (Schnitzer 1978), suggests that aphasia is an impairment of competence and that performance deficits (which he equates with deficits in particular modalities) cannot be regarded as genuine aphasia.

This argument becomes important for the clinician faced with the problem of deciding whether to introduce an alternative artificial communication system to a global aphasic patient. The work of Glass, Gazzaniga and Premack (1973), for instance, which reported that global patients were able to cope well with an artificial system made up of arbitrary shapes, would support the view that even in patients with global performance deficits, an underlying linguistic competence of some sort remains intact, but inaccessible. Such compensatory systems would appear to be accessing linguistic competence in by-passing impaired performance. The possible role of artificial languages in aphasia therapy is discussed in this volume by Rowley (chapter 15) and an application of one system is described by Bailey (chapter 16).

Jackson's (1874) distinction between the *propositional* (voluntary, meaningful) and *non-propositional* (automatic) language of aphasic patients also has implication for therapy. It was Jackson's view that non-propositional language is produced by the undamaged and uninhibited right hemisphere following left-hemisphere damage and it is often the only form of language available to the severe patient. Luria (1970), for example, discusses methods of shaping non-propositional automatic responses by progressing from automatic speech to propositional language, and Weigl (1961) has examined the phenomenon of temporary 'deblocking'. This deblocking method makes use of intact modalities and retained abilities to provide additional synaptic excitation to temporarily release blocked elements. Some of these techniques are not new, but the advantage of Weigl's method is that it is systematically applied and has a strong theoretical base.

It is Weigl's view that deblocking techniques can be applied to most forms of aphasic impairment thus demonstrating intact linguistic competence. In this volume Gielewski (chapter 12) and Huskins (chapter 11) respectively describe therapeutic methods for sensory deficits and expressive difficulties, based on the approaches advocated by Luria, which make use of patients' retained abilities.

The practical application of linguistic approaches to aphasia therapy might take advantage of the large pool of techniques and drills which have been developed in applied linguistics for second-language learning. Crystal, Fletcher and Garman (1976) provide a general discussion of the applications of some of these techniques in remediation. Patterson, Purell and Morton (chapter 6), in testing the efficacy of the traditional 'phonemic cueing' technique, have highlighted the necessity for such procedures to be carefully evaluated. The chapter by Hatfield and Shewell presents a number of linguistic approaches to aphasia therapy, which are worthy of careful empirical evaluation to determine their effectiveness.

A nonverbal perspective

There is more to human communication than its linguistic aspect and it is proposed that the other major semiotic system utilized in human interaction—nonverbal and paralinguistic behaviour—requires careful consideration by the aphasia therapist. This perspective on aphasia therapy is important for three main reasons. Firstly, it may be the case that an individual patient is impaired in his or her ability to use nonverbal communication, and the clinical decision may have to be taken to provide treatment in this area. Secondly, where a patient is unimpaired in this way of communicating, the therapist may feel that the retained abilities can be utilized and enhanced to aid communication. Whichever is the case, these aspects of communication need to be carefully assessed. Thirdly, it is important for the aphasia therapist to evaluate his or her own use of nonverbal communication in interacting with patients.

As a result of the research in this area in the last 10 years, it is now possible to catalogue a considerable number of nonverbal cues, all of which have perceptible effects upon communicative behaviour (Hinde 1972; Argyle 1975). In a recent book designed to help those in the interpersonal professions to study social skills, Hargie, Saunders and Dickson (1981) list nearly 20 different behaviours. They divide these into three categories; relatively rapidly-changing aspects of behaviour, relatively stable aspects of behaviour and paralanguage. The first category includes bodily contact, facial expressions, eye contact, head-nods and gestures. Included in the second category are a wider variety of cues which are more difficult to change during social interaction, such as body shape, hair, face, proximity, orientation and posture. Under paralanguage Hargie *et al.* include those vocal cues which can both assist understanding and convey emotion, such as pitch, tone, speed and volume.

Recently, there has been an increase of research into the role of nonverbal aspects of communication in aphasic patients. Goodglass and Kaplan (1963) in a classic study, investigated gesture and pantomime in aphasic patients. They concluded that there is a 'gestural deficiency which is best understood as an apraxic disorder consequent to a left-hemisphere lesion' (p. 719) and not as a general communication disorder. Recently Duffy and Buck (1979) have shown that the impaired pantomimic ability in aphasic patients correlates with severity of verbal deficit. However, this study also shows that these patients were unimpaired in their ability to communicate accurately using facial expression. Furthermore, in another study, Buck and Duffy (1980) found that aphasic patients were more expressive than either right-hemisphere damaged patients or controls in their nonverbal responses to emotive slides. Similarly, Boller, Cole, Vrtunski, Patterson and Kim

(1979) found that sentences with emotional content produced a greater number of responses than linguistically matched neutral sentences in aphasic patients. These studies provide further support for the general finding that the right hemisphere is responsible for processing the emotional and nonverbal aspects of language (Gainotti 1972; Ross and Mesulam 1979; Cicone, Wapner and Gardner 1980).

There have only been a few systematic attempts to apply the findings of studies of this type to treatment. Included in a broad approach to the treatment of mental disorder developed by Trower, Bryant and Argyle (1978), are a variety of methods for assessing and remediating nonverbal behaviour. Davis and Wilcox (1981) have advocated that therapy for aphasic patients should be directed at encouraging patients to communicate by using any available means. Gesture is an important component of their PACE programme (Promoting Aphasic's Communication Effectiveness). Similarly, Prinz (1980) has shown that aphasic patients are able to formulate requests if encouraged to use both verbal and nonverbal strategies. Schlanger and Freimann (1979) have demonstrated that pantomime therapy can generalize and further improve both pantomime expression and comprehension. Furthermore, Ostreicher (1980) has designed a gestural-verbal technique to help elicit verbal language. He suggests that it helps verbal communication and auditory comprehension.

What seems to emerge from the chapters by Rowley (15), Bailey (16), and Enderby and Hamilton (17), as well as the studies reviewed above, is that aphasic patients often exhibit a certain amount of resistance to the use of 'alternative' systems of communication. It would appear that they find some difficulty in accepting artifical languages, gestural systems and communication aids as alternatives to conventional speech. This may simply be a reflection of their unwillingness to accept that speech will never return. It may also be the case that there are other cognitive factors involved which may, for example, be related to concreteness of thought. However, this general interest is to be welcomed, but perhaps future research should focus much more on the use of supplements as therapeutic tools, for supporting rather than replacing speech.

A neuropsychological perspective

Aphasia, although an observable linguistic disorder, clearly constitutes a breakdown in neuropsychological processes and the cognitive mechanisms upon which language is dependent. Research in this area is providing new insights into the relationships between observable behaviour and underlying neurological correlates. Furthermore, the notions of neural-reorganization, inhibition and re-establishment, have particular relevance for those concerned with planning therapy, and may direct therapists to consider the related functions of associated undamaged brain sites and mechanisms and to use this information to the full in therapy.

From the therapeutic standpoint, it may be more useful to look beyond aphasia as a disorder of language *per se*, and to consider more closely the disrupted processes underlying its observable characteristics. Zangwill (1975) has noted that 'if [aphasia] is truly restricted to language then the patient should be at no greater disadvantage than a healthy individual endeavouring to communicate in a language with which he is imperfectly acquainted' (p. 96). In other words, it is clear that much more is involved at a cognitive level than an isolated impairment in linguistic ability, and Zangwill proceeds to discuss a number of nonverbal cognitive functions which are affected to some extent in aphasic patients. These include pantomime and gesture, musical ability, drawing and modelling, as well as tests of classification, abstraction and nonverbal intelligence.

A number of studies provide further support for the view that aphasic impairment constitutes a disruption in underlying neurocognitive functions. For instance, there are reasons to suppose that anomia in aphasic patients is a lexical access problem which is highly dependent upon perceptual-gnostic factors (Bisiach 1966; Tsvetkova 1975; Cohen and Keltor 1979) which suggests that there are problems in the actual identification of objects prior to lexical access and selection. Godwin (chapter 13) discusses the treatment of pure alexia (which is seen by many as a form of visual agnosia) through the systematic manipulation of the visual characteristics of the text, together with a facilitating use of phonic rules. A further indication of the importance of non-linguistic higher cortical functions is provided by Spinnler and Vignolo (1966) and Varney (1980), who found that language comprehension impairment in aphasic patients is closely related to impairment in environmental sound recognition.

In relationship to this issue, there has been much discussion concerning the extent to which Broca's aphasia can be considered an aphasia at all. The syndrome has been redefined in recent years as predominantly characterized by an apraxia of speech, that is, as a lower-level phonetic impairment due to faulty programming of initiation and/or coordination of articulation and phonation, rather than as a higher-level linguistic (syntactic or phonological) impairment. The discussion can be followed in Johns and LaPointe (1976), Buckingham (1979), Berndt and Caramazza (1980) and Code and Ball (1982).

That there should be impairments in non-linguistic cognitive functions in aphasic patients is hardly surprising given that the communicative process between speaker and hearer involves movement, perception and memory in many modalities. In planning therapy, therefore, full consideration should be given to the contribution of such underlying factors to an individual patient's particular difficulties. The relevance of neuropsychology to aphasia therapy is discussed in this volume by Purser (chapter 3) and an experimental application of theory and technique is described by Code (chapter 4). Hatfield (chapter 14) describes a therapeutic approach to aquired agraphia based on a neuropsychological explanation of the disorder.

A psychosocial perspective

It is something of a truism to say that aphasia causes not only difficulties in communication, but also massive psychosocial problems for patients and their families. Despite the fact that this goes unchallenged, little systematic effort appears to go into assessing these psychosocial problems and even less into therapeutic intervention. The psychosocial perspective in aphasia therapy is consequently the most under-developed. This probably stems from the notion of the aphasia therapist's traditional role as a 'speech' therapist solely concerned with observable linguistic deficits. However, it must be recognized that the fundamental aim of the aphasia therapist is the rehabilitation of the patient, and clearly psychosocial adjustment must constitute a major part of genuine rehabilitation. Furthermore, it may be the case that the degree of recovery which the patient makes in communicative abilities is closely related to the patient's level of psychosocial adjustment.

Psychosocial adjustment to aphasia entails coming to terms with a totally new set of circumstances, adjusting self-perceptions and perhaps adopting an entirely different role within the patient's social setting. The most widely used model for describing this process in stages is the 'grief' model of Kubler-Ross (1970) adapted with minor modifications by Sarno (1980a). There is a natural psychological resistance to unpleasant changes in life and sudden and traumatic handicap in a once healthy person is a devastating change. The everyday relationships human beings enjoy with others can contribute a great deal towards the quality of life. Any individual whose ability to foster and maintain relationships with loved ones, friends, colleagues and society as a whole is seriously disrupted, requires support, understanding and positive assistance. Clearly, the professional helper having the most intimate contact with the patient and the widest appreciation of the patient's problems is well suited to adopt this role. It is felt that as a general principle patients should not be discharged, even if their linguistic abilities have plateaued, while there are still outstanding problems in psychosocial adjustment.

There are then a number of factors concerning psychosocial adjustment which the aphasia therapist should take into consideration. Firstly, the psychosocial and emotional effects on the actual patient need careful evaluation and skilled intervention. Brumfitt and Clarke (chapter 7) present a psychotherapeutic approach to such problems in aphasic patients. Secondly, therapists need to become actively involved in monitoring the interpersonal factors affecting the patient, especially the role of relatives and others as shown by Müller and Code (chapter 8). Finally, therapy should be programmed to foster psychosocial adjustment, perhaps through the use of group treatment as discussed by Fawcus (chapter 9). Group treatment also constitutes a semi-naturalistic situation, a step nearer real-life, where an essentially social atmosphere may be used by the therapist to encourage interaction and the discussion of psychosocial problems. Meikle and Wechsler (chapter 10) report on the use of partly-trained volunteers and their work in the homes and with the families of aphasic individuals. This approach is clearly naturalistic and avoids confining therapy to traditional clinical settings. However, the ramifications of this kind of approach have yet to be established and David (chapter 2) discusses some of the problems in designing evaluative studies. Perhaps the greatest gain from a naturalistic approach is that a patient's everyday functional needs can best be identified, and realistic remediation undertaken to meet them.

A systematic behavioural perspective

It is proposed that the adoption of a systematic behavioural perspective to any treatment plan is more likely to produce positive results than an unstructured approach. Language is behaviour and aphasic language is disordered behaviour. The application of behavioural techniques to aphasia therapy is implicit in many remedial methods described in the literature as well as in this volume and aphasia therapists have been using such techniques, perhaps in an unstructured and intuitive manner, for a long time.

It would appear that the main value of a behavioural perspective may be that therapists can provide a systematic hierarchical framework for a treatment programme where targets (the required responses) can be specified in behavioural terms and materials and methods (the stimuli) can be chosen with care and utilized objectively. In this way treatment will start from a baseline which specifies, on the basis of naturalistic observations and the results of assessments, what the patient is actually capable of. This makes it possible to present material which has been graded into a hierarchy of discrete and easy targets. The systematic application of imitation and modelling, prompting and cueing and the use of appropriate positive reinforcement helps shape the patient's initial responses. Eventually this is followed by fading, and once the target behaviour has been acquired, and is occurring without assistance, therapy moves towards generalizing the behaviour into the patient's natural repertoire.

A behavioural perspective has been reported in a number of therapeutic approaches to aphasia. Examples can be seen in the highly specified programmed instruction approach adopted by Holland (Holland and Harris 1968; Holland 1970) and the computer-based methods suggested by Seron, Deloche, Moulard and Roussele (1980). At a more general level are the systematic hierarchial methods of training for melodic intonation therapy described by Sparks and Holland (1976) and the eight-step hierarchical approach for apraxia of speech described by Rosenbek, Lemme, Ahearn, Harris and Wertz (1973) and Deal and Florance (1978). The melodic intonation training programme, for instance, is broken down into four levels, each of which consists of a number of steps. Work moves up a level following a 90 per cent criterion of success at the preceding level. There is a gradual increase in the length of target utterances, a gradual fading of dependency on the therapist and of reliance on intonation. LaPointe (1977) has described a Base 10 format which can be adopted for many therapeutic programmes. This includes a printed form where therapeutic aims can be specified and baseline measures recorded. Progress in terms of behavioural criteria can be displayed graphically in order to provide reinforcement, in the form of feedback, for the patient and to enable a permanent record to be kept.

The utilization of behavioural techniques recognizes that an appreciation of the stimulus-response properties of therapeutic tasks should be automatic components of treatment programmes. This analysis is equally applicable to any consideration of psychosocial factors (Damon, Lesser and Woods 1979) and simply emphasizes the importance of the actual initial and target behaviours. It is suggested that practical intervention is heavily reliant upon the use of behavioural techniques and that these should be explicitly specified in treatment programmes before therapy commences.

An ongoing evaluative perspective

It is an axiom of aphasia therapy that useful treatment cannot proceed without assessment. The approach to therapy outlined here proposes that this axiom be extended to include ongoing evaluation parallel with the implementation of therapy. This implies that the clinician is constantly modifying and updating perceptions of the effects of treatment to take into account the progress made in each session on each task, and is not simply administering a standard battery once every three months. Ongoing evaluation can be seen as a process of hypothesis testing, resulting in the modification of existing hypotheses or the production of alternative hypotheses for testing. This implies that treatment programmes are not planned and carried out in a rigid manner, but that the patient's performance is the main determinant of the next step. The Base 10 procedure described above, for instance, allows for tasks to be modified according to whether progress is being made or not. The procedure can only increase the therapist's detailed knowledge of the patient's deficits, abilities and overall adjustment.

The usefulness of a number of standard aphasia-assessment batteries in forming a basis for treatment has been more fully discussed elsewhere (Müller, Munro and Code 1981). However, while most standard tests are good at classifying the patient in terms of aphasia type and severity, little attention has been given to establishing whether the patient can actually benefit from therapeutic assistance. Some batteries do allow the repetition of commands or minimal cueing (Porch 1971, Goodglass and Kaplan 1972) and imitation (Schuell 1965), or provide means whereby delayed responses can be reflected in the final scores; but performance produced with assistance is penalized. Furthermore, selective positive reinforcement is not permissable in administering standardized tests. From the point of view of rehabilitation, there is clearly a case for developing or adapting a battery which assesses the ability of the patient to benefit from the therapeutic techniques of reinforcement, modelling, shaping and fading, and to reflect this important ability in positive terms in the final score or profile. In addition, batteries which are designed in the future to help in planning therapy should attempt to assess a patient's ability to use compensatory nonverbal communication in a more comprehensive manner. Coltheart (chapter 18) describes a carefully designed hypothesis-testing method which can be applied with individual patients to test specific techniques.

Given the perspectives discussed in this chapter, it is desirable that assessment and ongoing evaluation should examine carefully the linguistic and underlying neurocognitive aspects of patients' problems, as well as their overall psychosocial adjustment. The observation has been made that existing aphasia batteries are linguistically inadequate (Lesser 1978; Whitaker and Whitaker 1979), and it has been suggested above that they are poor indicators of which therapeutic procedures to adopt. Furthermore, there are few readily available procedures to assess adjustment in common usage. A further danger of standardized tests is the inherent temptation to teach the test itself; a strategy which usually fails to result in generalization into the patient's everyday repertoire.

A more sensitive approach, and one which is particularly useful in evaluating single cases at a behavioural level, is the development of criterion-referenced profiles. With regard to syntax, for instance, the LARSP profile described by Crystal, Fletcher and Garman (1976) provides a useful and relatively simple method of describing a patient's grammatical abilities. Similarly, it may be possible to build up profiles for neurocognitive skills from various procedures which are described and reviewed in a number of places (Christensen 1974; Lezak 1976; Golden 1978; Walsh, 1978). The dearth of research into psychosocial aspects of aphasia means that the aphasia therapist has only limited guidelines for assessing adjustment, and it is hoped that more work will be developed along the lines of Mulhall (1978) and Müller and Code (chapter 8).

It is suggested that for therapeutic purposes the evaluation of a patient's problems should be a constant ongoing process incorporating a linguistic, nonverbal, neurocognitive, behavioural and psychosocial perspective. In order to attain this end, standard batteries need adapting and supplementing to take into account the specific requirements of the therapeutic situation. The uncertainty concerning the efficacy of aphasia therapy (David, chapter 2, and Coltheart, chapter 18) may be a reflection of the lack of appropriate and sensitive assessment procedures for the evaluation of individual patients, rather than a result of ineffective intervention strategies.

Conclusions

The foregoing overview of aphasia therapy is not intended to be prescriptive in pointing the therapist towards particular treatment methods or techniques. What has been suggested however is that any programme for treatment must be planned in terms of a linguistic and nonverbal perspective which recognizes that aphasia is caused by a disruption in brain behaviour relationships which constitute the underlying neuropsychological substrate of aphasia. Furthermore, psychosocial aspects of aphasia should no longer be considered secondary effects, but central, and naturalistic approaches should be examined more closely to determine their efficacy. It is also argued that therapy and its evaluation depend upon and benefit from a systematic behavioural perspective. In addition, a parallel hypothesis-testing approach to evaluation of an individual's problems in terms of the above factors should be built into the therapeutic programme.

There are many methods and approaches used in aphasia therapy, a range of which are discussed in this volume. Some are traditional yet relatively untested, while others have been systematically developed with strong theoretical foundations. This overview has tried to show, and the contents of this volume demonstrate, that linguistics, neuropsychology, psychotherapy and research methodology are inseparably combined in most approaches to aphasia therapy.

The professional whose concern is the rehabilitation of the aphasic individual—the aphasia therapist—must therefore be linguist, neuropsychologist, psychotherapist and researcher and should no longer view these perspectives on human behaviour as separate professional concerns, but as the necessary foundation of his or her therapeutic expertise.

Aphasia is a traumatic handicap and aphasia therapy has many unanswered questions. This volume does not provide all the answers, but it is hoped that it lays some foundations for future optimism for both patients and therapists.

The Efficacy of Aphasia Therapy

A dominating issue which has caused much discussion within aphasia therapy is whether it actually contributes towards the rehabilitation of the aphasic individual. The major obstacle to answering this question has been the problem of the design of research. David's chapter reviews the large-scale studies that have examined efficacy and outlines a study which attempts to overcome some of the problems. The reader can compare an alternative approach to the testing of efficacy which is discussed by Coltheart in the concluding chapter to this volume.

2

Researching into the efficacy of aphasia therapy

Rachel M. David

Introduction

Speech therapy for aphasia has a long history, dating from Broca's suggestion in 1865 that intensive and prolonged treatment would bring about a considerable improvement in the patient's condition. Since then, speech therapy has emerged and become established as a profession, and treatment programmes for all types of communication disorder have proliferated. It is only in the last 30 years or so that scientific attempts have been made to evaluate their effects. However, in Britain, the speech therapy service for adults is still developing and is unevenly distributed and generally understaffed. It is beset by many practical problems: various factors may limit the number of patients that can be seen and the intensity of treatment that can be offered; therapists often have a mixed caseload and are forced to weigh up the conflicting demands of different patient groups when planning treatment; in many areas there is still a lack of accommodation and equipment for the treatment of adult patients.

In 1975 two papers appeared which stimulated increased interest in the modes and evaluation of aphasia therapy. Hopkins (1975) suggested that there was no evidence in the literature to show that there was any basis to speech therapy other than the personal relationship established between therapist and patient. Similarly, Eaton Griffith (1975) reported the apparent success of a scheme for the treatment of aphasics based on general intensive stimulation by volunteers, which further demonstrated the importance of helping relationships in the management of aphasia. These papers, together with the practical difficulties involved in providing the service, resulted in the recognition by speech therapists of the need for careful investigations of their aims, techniques and effectiveness. Darley (1972a) had already posed the following questions which summarized the problems facing aphasia therapists: does therapy have a decisive influence on the course of recovery and the ultimate outcome; are the language gains attributable to therapy worth the necessary investment of time, effort and money; and what are the relative degrees of effectiveness of various modes of treatment of aphasia? In this chapter, previous attempts to answer these questions will be reviewed, and a current study which was designed to assess the contribution of non-specific encouragement to recovery from aphasia will be described.

Research review

In the papers to be reviewed in this chapter, the term 'speech therapy' in most cases implies some form of stimulation aimed at improving linguistic functioning. This is usually, but not always, undertaken by speech therapists. Linguistic stimulation is only one part of the speech therapist's role with aphasic patients, however, as it also includes assessment, counselling, social integration and help with adjustment to disability.

Although increased interest in the effects of aphasia therapy was stimulated by the papers referred to in the introduction, a few attempts at evaluation had been made prior to their appearance. Despite the relatively small number of reports overall, it is difficult to form any clear interpretation of their results in relation to the normal clinical situation. This difficulty arises mainly as a result of the large variations in method and design. These may be summarized under the following three headings; subject selection and control, assessment and treatment.

Subject selection and control

The design of aphasia therapy evaluation studies has progressed from large-scale retrospective surveys to smaller-scale studies of groups of carefully selected patients; the trend is now towards single-case designs (see Coltheart, chapter 18).

An early survey was that undertaken by Marks, Taylor and Rusk (1957), who studied 203 aphasic patients, 94 per cent of whom were stroke patients. 80 per cent of all the patients had been given language therapy in amounts of up to 110 sessions. 50 per cent had treatment for up to two months; 25 per cent had treatment for between 3 and 6 months. There was no formal control group. The outcome was expressed in terms of the amount of improvement shown on a four-point scale of 'excellent, good, fair' and 'poor'. About 50 per cent of the patients made fair to excellent progress. This study may be contrasted with one by Hagen (1973), in which 20 patients were the subjects of a stringently controlled research programme. The patients were selected on the basis of 13 strict criteria, including responses on the Schuell that would place them in Group III of that test, left posterior hemisphere lesions only, middle cerebral artery involvement only, lesion of an embolic or thrombotic origin, single lesion, no history of previous vascular episodes, and no history of alcoholism. These subjects were allocated to two groups, of which the first had speech therapy for one year (4 hours individual, 8 hours group and 6 hours independent work per week starting at six months post-stroke). The other group had all routine medical and non-medical services, but no speech therapy. Reassessment on the Schuell showed that only the treated group acquired functional reading comprehension, language formulation, speech production, spelling and arithmetic abilities. There was no difference between the groups in the recovery of auditory comprehension, auditory retention, visual comprehension or visual motor tasks.

Despite Hagen's careful research design and clearly presented results, it is difficult to apply them to a normal clinical situation. Few speech therapists have the amount of selection information available to them that this study demanded. Most of their patients are the elderly victims of, often, more than one stroke. This point was emphasized by Sarno (1976), who stressed that results from many evaluation studies are not readily generalized because of the unrepresentative age of the subjects alone. Unlike Hagen, few, if any, speech therapists can give as much as 18 hours a week of treatment to any patient. At the other extreme from Hagen's, the survey by Marks *et al.* was so unselective and loosely designed that the results are unclear and, hence, equally difficult to apply.

The importance of a control group is demonstrated by these reports. Studies which do not have a no-treatment group, or a group receiving an alternative form of treatment, have not proved very useful. Many investigators recognize this, but have difficulty in forming either a matched group or an equivalent one by random allocation of the subjects. The lack of comparable groups may spring from ethical doubts about withholding a treatment from some patients which might possibly be beneficial. However, this results in a paradoxical situation in which experimenters aim to establish scientifically whether a treatment is effective, whilst implicit in their research design is the belief that it *is* effective and therefore should not be denied any patient. The possibility that speech therapy might be harmful does not usually receive such consideration.

Vignolo and associates (Vignolo 1964; Basso, Capitani and Vignolo 1979; Basso, Faglioni and Vignolo, 1975) have undertaken a series of controlled trials of speech therapy. All of them have demonstrated some positive effects. Vignolo (1964) examined the records of 69 aphasic patients who had been tested twice, with a minimum interval of 40 days between the tests. Forty-two patients had had a minimum of 20 language therapy sessions over this period, with a minimum frequency of one session a week. Vignolo found no significant difference in progress between this group and the other 27 patients who were not treated. Basso *et al.* (1975) reviewed the progress of 185 aphasics to ascertain the effects of language rehabilitation on oral expression. Ninety-one of the patients were treated for at least 3 sessions a week for at least 6 months. The results indicated that treatment had a positive effect. Basso *et al.* (1979) investigated 281 aphasic patients, 162 of whom had had language rehabilitation. Treated patients were seen for no less than 5 months for at least 3 sessions a week. More patients in the treated group showed improvement in language skills.

It is an unfortunate weakness of these three studies that in each case the control group comprised patients who were too frail to tolerate treatment or were unable to attend for social or economic reasons. These are some of the very factors which might be expected to affect a patient's response to treatment. Darley (1975a) lists 10 such parameters which should be taken into consideration when selecting subjects for therapy-evaluation studies. They include the age, educational level, social status, prior language and non-language behaviour characteristics of the patient; the aetiology of the aphasia, its type and severity. An acceptable way to overcome the problem of matching this number of variables is by the random allocation of fairly large numbers of subjects to the treatment and/or control groups. This method has only recently come into use in evaluation studies. Meikle,

Wechsler, Tupper, Bennenson, Butler, Mulhall and Stern (1979) and Meikle and Wechsler (chapter 10, this volume) compared two groups of patients, randomly allocated, 16 having 'conventional speech therapy' and the other 13 volunteer treatment at home. No difference was found between the groups. Another study which used random allocation was undertaken by Wertz, Collins, Weiss, Brookshire, Friden, Kurtzke and Pierce (1978). A sample of 35 patients was given individual speech therapy and compared with a group of 32 patients given group language stimulation. Few significant differences appeared between the groups. The Wertz *et al.* study was a multicentre trial, a method of solving the general difficulty of acquiring adequate numbers of subjects which has not been used as often as might be expected, perhaps because of the considerable logistic problems which are involved.

Assessment

The choice of an assessment technique is central to the design of therapeutic evaluation studies, and the problem has been solved in ways which range from the rating scales of Marks *et al.* to the comprehensive test batteries of more recent workers. Numerous standardized aphasia tests are available, most of which are related to the theoretical bias of their authors. The two most widely used are probably the Boston Diagnostic Aphasia Examination (Goodglass and Kaplan 1972) and the Minnesota Test for the Differential Diagnosis of Aphasia (Schuell 1965).

The Boston test is a classificatory assessment, closely allied to theories of localization. It tests a wide range of communication skills, but the classification is done not so much on the results of the tests as on the basis of ratings of a sample of spontaneous speech. Aspects of communication which are rated are melodic line, phrase length, articulatory agility, grammatical form, paraphasia and word-finding. These aspects, together with the auditory comprehension scores, delineate profiles of distinctive shapes, into which approximately 75 per cent of patients may be categorized. It defines six major aphasic syndromes, namely: Broca's aphasia, Wernicke's aphasia, anomic, conduction, transcortical sensory, and transcortical motor aphasia. The Western Aphasia Battery (Kertesz and Poole (1974), is a modification of the Boston, classifying the patients on taxonomic principles into broadly the same groups, but with an 'Aphasia Quotient' as a measure of severity.

The Schuell is also an exhaustive assessment of most aspects of language. In 47 subtests it assesses behaviour under the headings of Auditory Disturbances, Visual and Reading Disturbances, Speech and Language Disturbances, Visuomotor and Writing Disturbances and Disturbances of Numerical Relations and Arithmetic Processes. Schuell used it initially to identify seven types of aphasia: simple aphasia, aphasia with visual involvement, mild aphasia with persisting dysfluency, aphasia with scattered findings compatible with generalized brain damage, aphasia with sensorimotor involvement, aphasia with intermittent auditory imperception and irreversible aphasic syndrome. Recent research using a cluster analysis of the test results of 86 patients, supports Schuell's later hypothesis of a severity-based classification system (Powell, Clark and Bailey 1979).

These tests, and most others, sample the modalities of communication and have mainly a pass/fail scoring system with the occasional use of scaled scoring for some subtests. The Porch Index of Communicative Ability (Porch 1967) developed the scaled scoring system to an advanced form with 16 parameters (e.g. Complex, Complete-delayed, Corrected, Cued, Unintelligible, etc.), and a patient can score from 1 (No Response) to 16 (Complex Response) for a given performance on a test task. Whilst adding greatly to the sensitivity of a test, the disadvantage of such a system is that its users require a high level of training. In this case 40 hours is recommended and frequent use of the test is essential for the maintenance of reliability.

A rather different approach to the assessment of communication is the investigation of functional performance. There have been few attempts to assess aphasic patients' spontaneous use of their residual language abilities. One test which examines this aspect is the Functional Communication Profile (Sarno, 1969). The FCP is based on an informal interview with a patient, after which 45 spontaneous communicative functions are rated on a nine-point scale. These scores can be converted into a percentage score which represents the proportion of the patient's previous communicative ability which has been retained. The test is subjective, based on the assessor's clinical appraisal of the patient's performance, but when used regularly by experienced clinicians has a high level of reliability (Sarno 1969). Results of interscorer reliability trials (David 1980) confirm this.

Problems of interpreting the results of speech therapy evaluation studies may arise from the use of these varied assessments. A test suitable for research is not always appropriate in the clinical situation, and it may be difficult for a clinician to compare the results of one test with another, and thus relate research results to the management of patients. However, the main interpretive difficulty is not so much in comparing the results of different tests as in relating them to the reality of the patient's condition. The question arises of whether a statistically significant change in the subtest scores of a formal assessment is reflected by a real change in the patient's conversational powers, in non-verbal communication skills or social adjustment. This is the problems of formal (diagnostic) versus functional (clinical) assessment. Formal assessments measure communicative performance in a test situation, but they may not depict a patient's communicative abilities in everyday activities, (e.g. shopping, etc.). Reinvang (1969) makes the point that to an aphasic, 'any situation demanding linguistic interaction is experienced as a test of his linguistic ability' (p. 112) and suggests that there is no sharp distinction between clinical and diagnostic performance.

Nevertheless, there have been few investigations of the aphasic's functional abilities as related to formal assessment results. Greenberg (1966) tested 50 aphasics on the FCP and the Schuell. Although there were many similarities, he found enough differences to justify separate testing with these two tests. Although Sarno, Silverman and Sands (1970) and Levita (1978) used the FCP as their major assessment in their evaluations of aphasia therapy, these studies lack the detailed information of a more comprehensive test. The former study was a comparison of the progress of three groups of global aphasics given either programmed treatment, non-programmed treatment or no treatment. Patients were tested on the FCP and on tasks which established their pre- and post-treatment level on the experimental programmes. There were no significant differences in outcome under the three treatment conditions. Levita investigated the progress of 17 patients given speech therapy as compared with 18 untreated patients from 4 to 12 weeks post-onset. No difference was found between the groups at 12 weeks, but the study may be criticized for its lack of pre-treatment assessments. Using the FCP and subtests of the Neurosensory Center Comprehensive Examination of Aphasia (Spreen and Benton 1969), Sarno and Levita (1979) studied 34 patients given speech therapy for 3 to 5 sessions per week for 11 months. Although patients improved on both tests, the change was statistically significant only on the FCP.

It can be argued that studies which have neglected to assess functional communication have ignored the main aim of aphasia therapy, which is to improve the quality of the patient's life by increasing communicative ability. Many of the studies referred to in this section have failed to provide adequate information on the progress of the patients because of incomplete assessment. Ideally, the subjects of such studies should receive a full diagnostic test as well as an assessment of their everyday communicative performance.

Treatment

A major difficulty in assessing the value of aphasia therapy is in defining the nature of the intervention. The term 'speech therapy', sometimes with the modifier 'conventional', is used to cover a multitude of approaches and techniques. Speech therapists themselves often have difficulty in defining their methods beyond the general description of their aims. This is probably because there are as many approaches as there are patients. Taylor (1964) describes many forms of non-specific stimulation undertaken in the name of therapy and Darley (1975a) outlines the two main direct approaches—stimulation and programmed instruction. The variety of approaches and their lack of definition are demonstrated by many evaluation studies which not only report inadequately on the nature of the treatment, but also fail to control its amount and duration. For example, Smith (1972) gave his subjects therapy for between 5 and 40 weeks with an average intensity of 25 hours per week. The procedures used were not described in detail, but were undertaken by graduate students. The interval between onset of aphasia and start of treatment was variable and patients were discharged when it was considered that their maximum improvement had been made.

This type of study raises two further questions with regard to treatment. Firstly, is therapy administered by partially or unqualified staff equivalent in its quality to that given by fully trained clinicians? Some investigators, such as Godfrey and Douglass (1959) who used occupational therapists to give language stimulation to their patients, show by the design of their research that they consider the nature of therapy not to be dependent on the professional qualifications of the therapist. Another opinion is that therapy by professional and non-professional personnel is not necessarily the same and that the possible differential effect should be examined. This viewpoint is exemplified by the study of Meikle *et al.* (1979; and chapter 10, this volume). They did, however, find no significant differences in the effects of therapy given by speech therapists and by volunteers. Secondly, the point at which patients are discharged from treatment in evaluation studies is important. Smith maintains that longer-term therapy is more effective, and Vignolo (1964) suggests that it should be continued for more than six months. But in both their studies patients were discharged when they had stopped making progress, many after less than six months of treatment. This throws the evidence for the effects of long-term therapy into some doubt. How many of the patients discharged earlier, for example, would have made further gains if they had been kept on for longer, and how many would have stayed the same or regressed?

In summary, it is important that the length of the post-onset interval at the start of treatment should be controlled. In addition, the amount, duration, quality and procedures of therapy should be defined and balanced between the treatment groups. Strict discharge criteria should be implemented whereby patients are discharged only after a certain amount of treatment, or when they have reached a predetermined level of communication. Some of these points are listed and discussed by Darley (1975a). These factors have been incorporated into the study described below.

The Bristol aphasia therapy evaluation study

A current evaluation of speech therapy for acquired aphasia is based in Bristol and investigates the hypothesis that recovery in aphasia may be a result of non-specific aspects of a helping relationship, rather than of professional therapeutic skills applied within that situation. It was designed to have more immediate relevance to the normal speech therapy clinic than had many previous studies. It is a multicentre trial, comparing the results of individual speech therapy with those achieved by untrained volunteers giving an equal amount of individual attention. There are 14 participating centres. All of the patients in the trial have been diagnosed by their referring doctor as having had a stroke. All of them are predominantly aphasic, although a mild degree of associated dysarthria is sometimes present. It was of great importance that the subjects should represent, as nearly as possible, the normal caseload of a hospital speech-therapy department. Therefore, such factors as advanced age or the severity of the communication disorder do not preclude enrolment. However, patients who are demented or who have sensory handicaps so severe that they are unable to cooperate with assessment, are excluded. Patients are also excluded if they are not English-speaking or have undergone previous speech therapy.

The assessments used in the trial are the Schuell and the FCP. The Schuell is a widely used test, the results of which are readily understood by practising speech therapists. The FCP is also fairly well known, and is a reliable assessment of functional communication. In combination, these two tests form a balanced battery which gives a comprehensive picture of clinical and diagnostic performance. Patients are assessed, using the FCP, at not less than three weeks post-stroke. A week later, they receive another assessment on both the FCP and the Schuell.

Immediately after this, they are randomly allocated to either a speech therapist or a volunteer for treatment.

Patients assigned to speech therapy receive individual treatment for approximately 2 hours a week for a period of between 15 and 20 weeks, with 30 hours of treatment in all. The amount of treatment and its duration were determined following a feasibility trial (David, Enderby and Bainton 1979) and are representative of normal clinical services. The speech therapists treat the patient using such techniques as training and experience suggest to be appropriate. Forms have been devised on which the aims of treatment and the amount of time spent working on them are recorded by the therapist (Enderby and David 1976). These will be analysed in relation to the changes found on reassessment. Patients allocated to volunteers receive the same amount of attention from untrained and undirected helpers. The volunteers are asked to encourage patients to communicate as well as possible. During the course of treatment, patients are assessed regularly on the FCP by an external assessor. A full assessment is made at the end of treatment with full follow-up tests three and six months later. If a patient attains an FCP score of 90 per cent or above on two consecutive occasions within the treatment period (this score implies near normality), treatment is stopped, although post-treatment assessments will be administered.

Several aspects of the design of this trial show the influence of the studies reviewed above. For example, the type of patient and the amount, duration and nature of treatment are all representative of the average clinical caseload and facilities. Patients are randomly assigned to their treatment type, and there are strict entry and discharge criteria—all patients receiving the same amount of treatment. Assessments are done by a therapist who never treats the patient, and both a functional and a diagnostic assessment are used. Patients are reassessed after a period without treatment to examine its long-term effects.

Discussion

There are few firm conclusions to be drawn from aphasia therapy evaluations to date, although there is general agreement that aphasia improves with treatment. It is not clear how much improvement may be expected, nor for how long progress is likely to continue. The patients who show the least improvement are the global aphasics who are past the spontaneous recovery period. This finding was most dramatically demonstrated by Sarno *et al.* in the study referred to earlier. However, global aphasics of more recent onset may show improvement. Sarno and Levita (1979) found global aphasics making significant gains during the second six months of treatment, this having been initiated at four weeks post-onset.

Very intensive therapy (18–25 hours per week) seems to be more effective than a more intermittent exposure. This is a finding not from one comparative study, but a conclusion which may be drawn by comparing the results of several studies. Hagen (1973) gave his patients 18 hours of treatment a week for a year and found significant improvement in many areas when he compared them with untreated controls. This study may be contrasted with Vignolo (1964) whose patients received a minimum of 20 sessions of therapy over not less than 40 days with a minimum frequency of 1 session a week. The patients appear to have received much less intensive treatment than did Hagen's. Vignolo found no significant differences between his treated and untreated patients. The continuation of treatment over a long period has been suggested to be of importance. The significance of this recommendation when it is made on the basis of studies in which patients are given varying amounts of treatment without stringent discharge criteria is dubious. However, Sarno and Levita (1979) have demonstrated the value of the second six months of treatment to their global aphasics.

The picture of the effects of treatment on the natural pattern of recovery is further confused by the finding that patients whose treatment is initiated early tend to make more progress than those who start later. This has been noted by many investigators, including Vignolo (1964) and Smith (1972). The finding is obviously related to the concept of 'spontaneous recovery'. Culton (1969) documented the spontaneous progress of 21 patients of varying aetiology, over an eight-week untreated period. Eleven of the patients, who were less than 30 days post-onset, made much more improvement on language and intellectual tasks than the remainder, who were at least 11 months post-onset. However, when interpreting evaluation studies, it is important to distinguish between change and outcome. It would seem natural for patients whose treatment is started later to show less change, as they have already passed through the spontaneous recovery period. The question is whether the outcome after treatment, *and at the same length of time after onset in each case*, is worse for the patients who started treatment later than for the rest. This question awaits fuller investigation.

The possibility that different treatment techniques may have differing effects on the pattern of recovery also awaits more detailed study. Whether speech therapy has a specific action on linguistic recovery, or whether improvement is largely the result of general intense stimulation and encouragement, is still not certain. Attempts to map the individual recovery pattern of the various language modalities from the results of studies to date, are not very profitable. Studies which examine this aspect are so diverse in the types of patient, the amounts and types of treatment and the measurements used, that it is impossible to summarize their findings adequately in a paper of this length. The most general agreement is about the relative effects of treatment on auditory comprehension and verbal expression. Many studies have shown that in treated patients, comprehension abilities make relatively good improvement compared with expressive abilities (Kenin and Swisher 1972; Lomas and Kertesz 1978; Prins, Snow and Wagenaar 1978; Basso *et al.* 1979; Sarno and Levita 1979).

Conclusion

In spite of the volume of research which has been undertaken, our understanding of the effects of treatment on acquired aphasia is still incomplete. There are two main reasons for this. Firstly, the fundamental structure of the disorder and its natural history when untreated is not fully defined or comprehended. This leads to an inevitable difficulty in interpreting the results of studies of the efficacy of treatment. Secondly, the majority of efficacy studies have shown methodological shortcomings and inconsistencies which give rise to difficulty in making comparisons between them. Their ambiguous results lead to a serious lack of clear information which would be of practical use to the aphasia therapist. Future work in this area should aim to provide the speech therapists who organize and carry out the service for aphasic patients, with information which would enable them to deploy their resources of time, personnel and expertise to the maximum benefit of the patients.

Neuropsychological Perspectives.

In the past neuropsychology's main concern has been to learn from pathology, but recent years have seen the development of a concern for a clinical application of theory and technique, not just for assessment, but also to therapy. In this section Purser assesses the application of neuropsychology to aphasia therapy and Code describes a study which attempts to apply recent research findings and experimental techniques from neuropsychology to treatment. The reader is referred also to the related chapters by Gielewski (12), Godwin (13), Hatfield (14), Rowley (15) and Bailey (16), all of which discuss some application of general neuropsychological knowledge and illustrate the growing importance of this field in aphasia therapy.

3

Therapeutic implications of neuropsychology

Harry W. Purser

Introduction

Neuropsychology, the study of the relationship between brain and behaviour, has undergone considerable revision since the pioneering work of the early neuroanatomists. At the turn of the present century neurologists encountered patients displaying a wide range of physical and psychological deficits following brain damage. The precise nature of this damage could only be determined at a postmortem examination. Psychology was similarly hampered by its prevailing methodological limitations. Introspection was the principle means of gaining access to the mind, which, in the case of aphasia, became redundant as a valid and reliable methodology. The consequence of these inherent limitations was minimal interaction between psychology and the neurosciences. A further general difficulty which dogged clinical workers in the field of brain damage concerned the inadequacy of available assessment procedures. Assessment of brain dysfunction relied on physical examination together with rather broad and vague observations of the extent to which mental functioning (including language) had been disrupted. Finally, the typical clinical population upon which the majority of early observations were made consisted of elderly patients suffering from degenerative conditions and cerebro-vascular accidents (CVA).

Against this background Pierre Broca (1861, 1865; see Kraetschmer 1981, for a review) advanced one of the first anatomical explanations of aphasia through his observation that damage to the third frontal gyrus of the left hemisphere was invariably associated with deficits in verbal expression. He concluded that this cortical site was responsible for the motor patterns of speech. A few years later Wernicke (1874; see Eggert, 1981, for a review) advanced a more comprehensive model of language impairment following brain injury; here, in addition to Broca's area, a further site on the first temporal gyrus of the left hemisphere was identified, damage to which led to difficulties in the comprehension of spoken language. Wernicke's conception of brain function hinged on the idea that the brain is physically organized in such a way that different regions process specific kinds of information which are then integrated by 'association areas' to culminate in a continuous interchange between brain and external environment. Aphasic arrest could be the result of damage to specific processing centres or through damage to the interconnecting pathways between these centres. Each type of damage would lead to consistent patterns of deficits and thus Wernicke's model was essentially predictive; it could specify what patterns of deficit would be likely to arise if certain brain regions were damaged. Further, given a particular cluster of symptoms the model could be used to deduce where brain damage was likely to have occurred without resorting to physical inspection of the cerebral cortex.

Within a few years a burgeoning literature developed which was dedicated to further speculation and theorizing on more complex models based on this 'localizationist' position on brain function. One major drawback to this endeavour lay in the often very subjective accounts of deficit patterns supplied by clinicians which made comparisons between studies highly unreliable. This inadequacy was particularly pertinent in aphasiology given the complexity of language deficits. There was a need for more objective and hence more reliable methods of describing and quantifying clinical syndromes if a valid system of classification was to develop which would allow direct comparisons between studies.

As psychology began to relinquish its reliance on introspection and move towards the more objective methods of Behaviourism the study of aphasia received renewed attention. The development of the 'mental test' by Binet and Simon (1905) provided new horizons for the clinical study of aphasia through the provision of objective methods for detecting and describing neuropsychological dysfunction. The beginnings of modern neuropsychology were laid during this period with an emphasis on the assessment of psychological dysfunction following brain damage and the production of theoretical models of brain function which related neuroanatomical damage to the resultant psychological deficits. This movement was based on several prevailing assumptions in medicine and psychology. Mental experience (consciousness) was seen as the product of neurophysiological activity; damage to neural tissue would therefore result in consistent and predictable symptom patterns. One further assumption was made about brain damage. Since neurophysiological damage is irreversible the physical and psychological deficits resulting from brain injury would be permanent consequences of brain damage. Such a view naturally offered a gloomy prognosis for the brain-damaged patient; rehabilitation was likened to caring for a mentally retarded amputee rather than as an active process aimed at the restoration of lost functions.

The flavour of neuropsychology during this phase was essentially academic. Brain-injured patients were studied in order to catalogue the range of deficits that could occur and to develop theoretical models of brain function which would illuminate normal mental processes. Here the abnormal was studied in order to infer how normal processes operate in the intact brain.

The impact of two major world wars rapidly changed the face of neuropsychology as new technological developments led to more powerful investigative procedures in the neurosciences. A further consequence was the emergence of a completely new population of brain-damaged patients; head injuries to young soldiers revealed a more dynamic constellation of symptoms which typically showed gradual improvement with the passage of time. This evidence was also underlined by the development of the new specialism of paediatric neurology where it was evident that even extensive brain damage in infancy could have a rather good prognosis, particularly for the development of language. By the 1950s it was clear that the age at which brain damage was incurred was a crucial prognostic variable.

New technology had greatly improved the clinician's ability to localize brain damage *in vivo* and further refinements in psychometric assessment procedures began to produce much more sensitive indices of deficit. A further landmark achievement occurred in the late 1950s when Penfield and Roberts (1959) demonstrated how surface electrical stimulation of the cerebral cortex could be used to 'map' psychological functions such as memory, speech and language. These techniques, together with advances in radiological visualization of the brain, produced increasingly detailed evidence of individual pathology.

By this stage neuropsychologists had produced several competing models of brain function. The early localizationist models had been refined and developed in the light of a growing body of clinical evidence, despite fundamental objections from the 'holist' school of neuropsychology. This latter movement argued that no simple one-to-one relationships existed between specific brain regions and discrete psychological functions (Head 1926; Lashley 1929). Holists argued that neural tissue acts *en masse* to perform complex higher mental operations and could therefore withstand limited local damage without serious deficits in functioning. When extensive damage did occur the functional system suffered a *general* rather than any *specific* deficit.

One further distinctive school of neuropsychology emerged in the USSR which was based on a very detailed *functional analysis* of psychological deficits and proposed that rather than specific brain structures being involved in language there were diverse brain regions responsible for various components of psycholinguistic processing. Luria (1970) outlined a model of brain function based on these principles which offers a further explanation for the recovery of function in aphasia. When a particular brain region is damaged there will be a loss of that portion of psycholinguistic function subserved by that region. In Luria's model recovery of function is achieved by related areas of tissue taking over the particular function of the damaged region.

By the 1960s neuropsychologists were immersed in applying the new concepts of computer technology to the modelling of brain function (Miller, Galanter and Pribram 1960). This approach, of making an analogy between the brain and a sophisticated computer, has generated abstract models of neuropsychological processes which do not necessarily have any physical counterpart in neural tissue. Rather, neuropsychologists attempted to simulate such higher mental functions as language by actually programming computers to mimic communicative functions (Newell, Shaw and Simon 1961). Such studies provided a rich source of theoretical ideas which other branches of the neurosciences could attempt to translate into neural and clinical terms. This new class of representational models has drawn heavily on the transformational-generative grammar approach to linguistics resulting in a new breed of brain scientist—the neurolinguist. Here aphasic syndromes are viewed as consistent patterns of errors generated by disruption of normal psycholinguistic processing as illustrated by the work of Kean (1978), Meyerson and Goodglass (1972) and Schuell and Brewer (1969).

Despite this new sophistication in the analysis of deficits in aphasic syndromes, the notion of localization of function has held intuitive attractiveness for many workers and can be seen in modified form in the recent account of aphasiology given by Geschwind (1969; 1970; 1979). Here, in addition to the areas identified by Broca and Wernicke, Geschwind postulates one further area in the inferior parietal lobe which mediates cross-modal associations such as the integration of auditory stimuli (words) with the sensory properties of the objects these stimuli represent. This ability is supposedly species-specific and is the basis of the capacity for object naming in man. Geschwind's model goes further in specifying the complex pathways that must exist if the diversity of deficit syndromes seen in aphasia are to be explained.

One further feature of Geschwind's model deserves consideration; he stresses the existence of multiple pathways which could account for a number of atypical aphasic presentations and form the basis of his account of recovery of function following brain damage. The model postulates that several pathways may exist which convey information between the various processing sites. Of these pathways it is assumed one is the most efficient channel of intracerebral communication, but in the event of its destruction alternative pathways can continue to relay the information, although with varying degrees of relative efficiency.

Evidence for the localization of function

Although localization models seem intuitively to offer the most parsimonious accounts of brain injury, the evidence upon which these models have been based now seems rather sparse. Penfield and Roberts (1959) are often cited as having provided definitive examples of the localization of speech functions. Close inspection of their work reveals that they were unable to establish any particular site in the left hemisphere which, in general, resulted in aphasic arrest. Rather it seemed that any gross stimulation of the left hemisphere could result in varying degrees of speech disturbance. Lenneberg (1974), in a review of the available evidence of localization of speech, concluded that no structurally well defined areas could be identified which were consistently associated with clinical language deficits. At best one could postulate 'gradients of probability' which might relate a lesion site with a particular symptom complex.

A further source of evidence often invoked for the localization of language concerns the observation that only Man has the capacity for symbolic communication. Here it is suggested that the various swellings and bulges in the cortical lobes represent evolutionary developments which make symbolic communication possible. This view, however, has been seriously undermined by the work of Gardener and Gardener (1969) and Premack (1971) in their demonstration of symbolic communicative capacities in primates.

Yet even when specific cortical sites are questioned there remains the more general proposition that the existence of marked asymmetries of function between the two hemispheres is highly suggestive of distinct, anatomical specialization. The consistent finding that the left hemisphere specializes in linguistic processing whereas the right is concerned with non-verbal (spatial) processing has stood since the time of Broca and has received powerful support from a revolutionary series of observations by Sperry (1966; 1970). In order to relieve intractable epilepsy the main bundle of interconnecting fibres between the two hemispheres (the corpus callosum) was cut, resulting in the 'split-brain' phenomenon. This *commissurectomy* procedure virtually isolates the two hemispheres (although subcortical interconnecting pathways are spared) since inter-hemispheric information exchange is abolished. Despite the radical nature of this surgery it is very difficult to detect any obvious psychological deficit following recovery from surgery.

However, when sensitive psychological assessments are carried out a distinct pattern of dysfunction emerges. Gazzaniga (1970; 1975) likens the resultant functioning to having two completely independent minds, each capable of perceiving, memorizing and performing operations when information is deliberately restricted to each hemisphere. This type of restricted input can be achieved by blindfolding patients and having them identify common objects placed in each hand. Objects manipulated by the right hand are processed by the left hemisphere and vice versa. A further method makes use of the special anatomical arrangement of the visual pathways in the brain in order to restrict visual input to one or other hemisphere. This can be achieved by use of the tachistoscope—a device which can briefly illuminate visual stimuli for a variety of time settings. By devising visual arrays which consist of left and right visual field stimuli, and having a central fixation point, it is possible to deliver the information in the right visual field to the left hemisphere, and information on the left to the right hemisphere. Tachistoscopic presentation briefly exposes discrete messages to each hemisphere allowing the neuropsychologist to compare the efficiency of each hemisphere with different types of input. A similar effect can be accomplished for auditory stimuli by the use of dichotic listening tests. Discrete stimuli can be presented simultaneously to either hemisphere by the use of stereophonic headphones. See Code (chapter 4) for further detailed description of these techniques and their application in rehabilitation.

Using these techniques it was observed that the mental capabilities of the two hemispheres were not symmetrical. When an object was presented to the left hemisphere (either manually or visually) patients could supply its name either verbally or through written language. In contrast, objects presented to the right hemisphere could not be named, although patients could often manipulate the item appropriately, demonstrating non-verbal processing was possible in the right hemisphere.

These experiments, together with the majority of clinical observations of aphasia, resulted in a seemingly definitive view of the left hemisphere as the seat of language capacities. The right hemisphere was relegated to processing spatial information and the comprehension of very simple linguistic input. In addition to this dichotomy of linguistic/spatial processing in the hemispheres it was suggested that further asymmetries might exist. Although much of the evidence is anecdotal, Sperry (1966) and Dimond (1979) refer to what appears to be the existence of two 'personalities' in split-brain patients where the left hemisphere mediates laughter and humour and the right displays more sombre and depressive tendencies.

This initial picture of a marked division in consciousness has been revised in the light of work by Milner (1974) and Zaidel (1973; 1974; 1978). Milner, in the course of her series of temporal lobectomies for the relief of epilepsy, has provided data suggesting that language specialization is not always the province of the left hemisphere, even in well established right-handed patients. A proportion of patients seem to have a fairly equal collaboration between the hemispheres in linguistic processing. Zaidel, using further specialized experimental procedures, has been able to demonstrate a far wider range of verbal abilities in the right hemisphere of split-brain patients than had been elicited in the earlier studies. These findings, together with a growing awareness that even within the left hemisphere it is difficult to identify specific anatomical sites where damage invariably leads to recognized aphasic syndromes (Ojemann and Whitaker 1978a; 1978b) have brought the notion of anatomical localization of speech and language functions into question. Contemporary neuropsychology therefore recognizes the variability in performance that can be encountered in brain-damaged patients, even when such damage is confined to relatively discrete neural regions.

Despite the advances in modern technology which have allowed very accurate diagnosis of cerebral pathology and precise localization of anatomical damage, it would seem that, at best, only probabalistic statements can be made about the functional significance of specific brain injury. Whereas psychological assessment of brain dysfunction has in the past contributed to the localization of damage, it is clear a new role is emerging for neuropsychological assessment. In the same way far reaching implications emerge for neurolinguists who have tried to describe the classic aphasic syndromes in linguistic terms. This quest to uncover the syntactic, semantic and phonological errors which might characterize the various clinical syndromes of aphasia has proved extremely difficult. Both Goodglass (1968) and Farmer and O'Connell (1979) have acknowledged the slow progress to date. The search for a universal 'grammar of aphasia' through the minute analysis of aphasic language performance has not, as yet, uncovered any specific and systematic patterns of disability in any of the aphasic subgroups. As Marshall (1973) has argued,

> the search for generality in the study of brain mechanisms is no doubt laudable—but it seems more likely that a theory of individual differences is a necessary prerequisite for success in this enterprise. Such a theory would specify how different subjects set up different representations of the strange tasks that neuropsychologists set them.
> (p. 467)

From theory to therapy

For many clinicians involved in the rehabilitation of brain-injured patients these interminable debates between rival schools of neuropsychological theory often fail to capture the imagination. It would seem that the most relevant issue, namely what can be done for these patients, is not being addressed. Indeed these debates have paid little more than lip service to the notion of active treatment for such patients; in consequence, a wide variety of stimulation techniques have developed in speech-therapy clinics which can really only claim face validity rather than being based on specific theoretical systems. As Thompson (1978) concluded in his recent review of trends in neuropsychology,

> there has been too ready an acceptance of deficits as permanent facts about a person, rather than as difficulties which might possibly be overcome by an energetic application of psychological principles. Stroke patients with speech disorders rarely have a psychologist to assist them, and still receive therapy for which it has proved difficult to find evidence of efficacy. Neuropsychologists have equally been too ready to rely on paper and pencil tests, rather than closely observing the patient under his normal working conditions. (p. 96)

The value of theory in any endeavour rests in its reliance on empirical testing to generate new hypotheses which can lead to further theoretical refinements. In the field of aphasia therapy several theoretical models can be identified which have more or less specific implications for rehabilitation. The complex models of the representational school often leave clinicians scratching their heads for practical applications, whilst the less specific formulations offer little more than very general guidelines for therapy. As Thompson points out, standard laboratory assessment batteries fail to simulate and capture the real problems experienced by the brain-injured patient. Whilst these forms of assessment may yield greater resolution on a particular pattern of dysfunction and serve as indispensable baseline measurements in the course of treatment evaluation, they can often seem trivial and irrelevant from the patient's point of view.

In recent years these criticisms have resulted in a more realistic and naturalistic approach to rehabilitation. The very fact that a great many patients do make very good recoveries from cerebral lesions has attracted considerable attention in the last five years. The remainder of this chapter will discuss various ideas that have been advanced to account for the recovery of function and outline new developments in rehabilitation which neuropsychologists are currently pursuing.

Recovery of function

Powell (1981) has reviewed the current paradigms available in neuropsychology which have generated several distinct positions on the recovery of function. He identifies three basic models—physiological, structural and process explanations.

1 Physiological models

(a) Diaschisis. This refers to the observation that damage to a particular area of brain tissue can result in the raising of firing thresholds in surrounding tissue. The implication is that initially there will be extensive but temporary reductions in function after a lesion. As diaschisis subsides so functions reappear in the brain-damaged patient.

(b) Regeneration. Although true regeneration is only seen in the peripheral nervous system some evidence suggests a comparable phenomenon may occur in the central nervous system. Much of this evidence comes from comparative animal studies which raises questions as to its relevance to man.

(c) Collateral sprouting. Here it is suggested that axons surrounding a lesion may send new dendrites into the damaged area which gradually replace the loss of neural tissue.

(d) Relatively ineffective synapses. This refers to the possibility that multiple pathways exist which can be utilized to re-route intra-cerebral information after damage to the principal pathways.

The difficulty with all these physiological explanations is twofold: first, the evidence upon which they are based is, by and large, rather slender; second, these explanations seem only to account for the initial, post-trauma recovery, which owes much to medical intervention and the brain's own biological defence systems.

2 Structural models

(a) Redundancy. Laurence and Stein (1978), among others, have argued that the brain has much more tissue devoted to specific psychological functions than is strictly necessary for efficient processing. In the event of damage it is this built-in redundancy which copes with new processing demands and ensures continuing adaptive functioning.

(b) Levels of representation. Implicit in the work of Luria (1966; 1970) lies the notion of hierarchical organization where the different layers of cortical tissue process incoming information in characteristic ways. Rosner (1974) contends that it is this multi-level representation of brain function which allows adaptation to injury through lower levels taking over the processing usually carried out by higher levels.

(c) Multiple control. This model postulates a number of neural 'centres' which effectively control specific psychological functions. Damage to a particular centre is therefore offset by the availability of 'back-up' centres which can continue to regulate that function.

Whilst structural models may offer a more credible account of longer term recovery of function they remain rather untestable hypotheses. If such systems do exist in neural tissue it almost seems that the mystery to be solved is why there should be any loss of function in the first place.

3 Process models

(a) Functional substitution. In this account it is argued that brain damage results in permanently impaired functioning, but that other functional systems can be employed to process task input. A simple example might be where damage to the auditory system can be minimized by the development of more sophisticated visual processing in order to lip-read. Here, *adaptation* to a specific deficit is advocated rather than any recovery of lost function *per se*.

(b) Plasticity. This notion has been quoted as an explanation of recovery of function in both children and adults (Stein, Rosen and Butters 1974). It is assumed that a new brain area can take over a damaged function since it may be developmentally 'primed' to do so. An example of this type of explanation is often given when considering the good prognosis for language development in children who have suffered extensive damage to the left hemisphere. During the early stages of language acquisition it is suggested that both hemispheres are equally involved in the processing of input and control of output. This early 'priming' of the non-dominant hemisphere facilitates the development of language capabilities when the dominant hemisphere sustains injury. Lorber (1980) has reported several follow-up cases of childhood hydrocephalus where perfectly normal psychological functioning is observed despite the fact that CAT scanning reveals only a few millimetres of neural tissue distributed around the inside of the skull! Such dramatic evidence of plasticity of function is rarely encountered.

(c) Reorganization of the processing flow. Luria contends that brain damage does not necessarily disrupt an entire functional system (Luria 1963, Luria, Naydin, Tsvetkova and Vinankaya 1969). Since a given functional system may be made up of complex interactions between topographically distant sites a specific lesion may only affect one particular sub-system. By careful analysis of the disturbed function Luria tries to isolate the specific subsystem deficit involved and programme treatment to establish new, more efficient subroutines which can 'fill in' for the lost subcomponent.

Process models perhaps hold out the most concrete suggestions for neuropsychological therapy although they range in their specificity from the relatively narrow approach of the functional substitution model to the rather global implications of the plasticity model. Luria's model perhaps holds the key to a science of recovery of function. The detailed analysis of the deficit pattern to establish both the exact nature of the loss and provide a treatment baseline offers the best hope of unequivocal treatment evaluation.

In contrast to the above models a completely different and more gloomy account of recovery of function is discussed by LeVere (1975; 1980). This thesis questions the fundamental effect of brain injury and is highly critical of the notion of 'recovery' of function. LeVere contends that a major component of the behavioural deficits following a brain lesion is due to the attempt to compensate for what may be temporarily inhibited functioning. Compensation then is the antithesis of recovery from brain injury and thus efforts must be made to minimize compensation if recovery of function is to be maximized. This point of view receives support from a number of animal experiments but as yet there are little human data to even begin to evaluate the position in a scientific manner.

Aphasia therapy

Having briefly outlined some of the major theoretical positions on the recovery of function we now move to consider more specific implications for aphasia therapy. Examination of typical recovery curves for aphasic patients reveals an initial period of rapid improvement within the first six months followed by a more gradual recovery to a plateau at the end of the first year (Vignolo 1964). It seems plausible that this initial phase of recovery could owe much to the stabilization of damage where physiological mechanisms play a crucial role. Thereafter structural or processing changes may account for further improvements.

If we accept a basic position that the potential for recovery of function is available within the brain, it remains to establish whether this process can be accelerated and enhanced through specific therapeutic techniques. Kertesz and McCabe (1977) have reviewed the prognosis of different aphasic subgroups and commented on the apparent efficacy of therapy for these groups. It would appear that in their sample there was little evidence to suggest that traditional speech-therapy techniques affect the eventual outcome. This study was however unable to specify in any detail exactly what these techniques were; as Darley (1972a) bemoaned earlier, the state of treatment evaluation in aphasia is often too confounded by inadequate methodology to arrive at any reliable conclusions. Holland (1975), in repeating this criticism, made a plea to aphasiologists to improve the quality (and quantity) of their research designs in order to minimize equivocal conclusions in therapy-evaluation studies.

Whilst this fundamental problem continues to haunt much of the nomothetic research in this area, there is a trend towards the use of experimental single-case methodology in therapy evaluation which cannot fail to enhance research in aphasia therapy. By the careful translation of neuropsychological theory into clinical therapy it will be possible to enrich the study of aphasia at both theoretical and practical levels. Before moving to a consideration of recent research findings it is worth outlining several major models of neuropsychological treatment which currently influence clinical practice.

1 Verbal conditioning

Goodkin (1969) demonstrated how systematic verbal reinforcement and punishment could improve the language output of a 56-year-old male patient who presented both sensory and motor aphasia with considerable word-finding difficulties. This patient was considered at his 'peak' of recovery two years post-trauma and had been discharged from therapy prior to the single case study. Goodkin was able to demonstrate a significant improvement in communicative ability after several months of treatment. Sarno, Silverman and Sands (1970) extended this treatment approach by using programmed learning to help teach new language patterns to aphasics.

2 Neuropsychological reorganization

Luria (1963) advocates the need to make a detailed assessment of which abilities have been disrupted within a particular cognitive function and then teach these abilities in order to 'fill in' the 'missing links' in the functional system. By directing specific stimulation at encouraging the formation of new subroutines it may be possible to develop new routes for carrying intracerebral information between primary, secondary and tertiary cortical areas.

3 'Preventive' technique

Beyn and Shokhor-Trotskaya (1966) concentrate on how the aphasic brain develops strategies for re-learning language. Here, some forms of aphasia are regarded as secondary to primary disturbances such as the reduction of generalization and abstraction capacities—resulting in telegraphic speech. This tendency to telegraphic speech can be prevented by very rapid post-trauma intervention (within first month) aimed at discouraging object-naming activities in order to encourage later grammatical performance.

4 Self-instruction strategies

Berman and Peelle (1967) stress the need to make the best possible use of residual capacities in order to foster the development of alternative processing strategies. Rather than address the known areas of deficit the patient is encouraged to devise and accumulate a series of strategies which make use of existing strengths.

5 Artificial language systems

Glass, Gazzaniga and Premack (1973) and Gardner, Zurif, Berry and Baker (1976) discuss the use of visual communication systems as a rapid method of restoring communicative functioning in aphasia. These approaches emphasize the value of prosthetic devices for severely handicapped patients rather than a genuinely therapeutic paradigm. (See Rowley, chapter 15, for further discussion.)

6 Minor hemisphere therapies

Sparks and Holland (1976) describe a procedure which provides a melodic vehicle for the aphasic patient with expressive difficulties. Here the assumption that the spatial talents of the right hemisphere can be utilized in language rehabilitation is tested through the use of melody (Melodic Intonation Therapy) to improve communicative functioning in severe expressive aphasia. The directed stimulation paradigm of Buffery (Buffery 1977; Buffery and Burton, 1982) is a further attempt to tap the inherent language capacities of the minor hemisphere by structuring therapeutic input in accordance with the known facts of hemispheric asymmetry. By utilizing the tachistoscope, dichotic listening apparatus and manual tasks it may be possible to selectively stimulate the right hemisphere to 'take over' linguistic processing, and Code (chapter 4) describes an experiment designed to examine this possibility.

Such therapeutic strategies are based on distinct models of brain function ranging from modified localizationist positions to holistic equipotentiality theories. In the former, particular emphasis is placed on the role of the right hemisphere in recovery of function and a growing body of research work supports the notion that the minor hemisphere plays a crucial role in the recovery process. Searleman (1977) in an extensive review of right-hemisphere linguistic capacities concluded that there was convincing evidence of language capacities transferring from the damaged left hemisphere to the intact right hemisphere. In some cases it was observed that further damage to the right hemisphere resulted in a second period of aphasic arrest.

A number of studies have highlighted the importance of the minor hemisphere in recovery from aphasia. Smith (1966) reported the case of a 47-year-old man who underwent dominant hemispherectomy for the removal of a glioblastoma. Following surgery, the patient displayed a severe receptive and expressive aphasia. Over a period of seven months language abilities showed steady improvement, and thus it was concluded that the minor hemisphere, inescapably, must have been responsible for this recovery of function. Pettit and Noll (1979) studied a group of 25 aphasic adults using dichotic verbal tests over a period of two months. As language abilities improved in these patients, so cerebral dominance (as measured by ear preferences) was seen to shift from the left to the right hemisphere. Cummings, Benson, Walsh and Levine (1979) also report a single case study of a 54-year-old man presenting aphasia through embolic infarction in the distribution of the left middle cerebral artery. Computerized axial topography revealed the destruction of the classic left-hemisphere language areas. As recovery of function progressed over a three-year period it was concluded that the minor hemisphere had been responsible for improvement. Czopf (1979) discusses a study of 22 aphasic patients who underwent intracarotid barbiturate injections to the right hemisphere (see Wada and Rasmussen, 1960, for further discussion of this procedure) in order to establish cerebral speech dominance. In the majority of cases this technique revealed right-hemisphere dominance although there were considerable individual differences in the sample. Such findings were seen as consistent with the notion that the right hemisphere can take over linguistic processing when the left hemisphere sustains severe damage.

In view of these findings, it would seem worthwhile to systematically explore how this process of dominance shift could be accelerated and made more efficient through structured therapeutic intervention. A starting point would be the recognition that in both normal and abnormal populations cerebral dominance for speech and language processing is seldom an all or nothing phenomenon. Given the considerable variability seen in clinical populations with similar anatomical lesions it may be the case that language dominance ranges on a continuum from left to right with the majority of individuals displaying left-hemisphere specialization.

Powell (1981) has recently offered a blueprint for the scientific investigation of neuropsychological therapy. From the outset he advocates regarding treatment as an *experimental* undertaking which emphasizes the need to employ single-case-study methodology in order to demonstrate the effectiveness of the particular therapeutic intervention being employed. (See Yule and Hemsley 1977, for discussion of single-case method and Coltheart, chapter 18). Powell's 'Brain Function Therapy' also stresses the need for detailed assessments of the individual patient in order to analyse psychological deficits and formulate specific behavioural goals for intervention from the very beginning of treatment. These measurements, together with physical investigations of cerebral damage, provide baseline information prior to treatment against which therapy effects can be compared. Finally, these initial assessments may have organic implications which can guide the therapist in designing specific remedial tasks aimed at achieving the stated therapy goals. Powell advocates a directed stimulation approach as suggested by Buffery (1977) utilizing appropriate techniques to deliver input to chosen brain regions in order to facilitate processing activity, but see Code (chapter 4) concerning some of the problems. This approach views the existence of individual differences in the functional localization of language as a good indication for neuropsychological therapy. The fact that Ojemann and Whitaker (1978b) have discovered differences in the cerebral localization of languages in bilingual patients may suggest that slight changes in the pattern of coding and encoding of language could change the topography of linguistic processing. Clearly this would have far-reaching implications for clinicians.

Powell's conception of Brain Function Therapy is similar to the approach of Keenan (1979) and Darley (1975b) where structured treatment includes the statement of goals in specific behavioural terms, and progress towards these goals is achieved in step-wise fashion suited to the needs of each individual patient. If such a rigorous methodology was adopted more widely in clinical practice there would be steady progress towards unravelling the enigma of recovery of function.

New directions

Neuropsychology continues to probe deeper into the mysteries of brain function and self-consciousness. Technological developments have dramatically increased the reliability of clinical diagnosis of brain damage *in vivo*; neuropsychological assessments provide sensitive indices of behavioural deficits and allow clinicians to define treatment goals before the commencement of therapy. New technological developments offer the clinician the opportunity to observe the effects of intervention 'on line'.

1 Regional cerebral blood flow (rCBF)

Lassen, Ingvar and Skinhøj (1978) describe a new technique for observing functional localization in the brain based on the fact that the flow of blood through the tissue of the body varies with the level of metabolism and the functional activity in those tissues. Thus the functional activity of neural tissue can be directly visualized by injecting a radioactive isotope into the main arteries of the brain which is then measured by an array of scintillation detectors. The information arriving at these detectors is then processed by computer and displayed on a colour television monitor where different hues represent different flow levels.

Soh, Larsen, Skinhøj and Lassen (1978) have explored the functional activity of the cerebral hemispheres in aphasic patients during speech acts and have observed a number of intriguing phenomena. Lassen *et al.* (1978) describe the activation of the minor hemisphere during speech in normal subjects. Although it is difficult to say what this global activation may mean such a finding at least suggests the minor hemisphere is very much involved in normal linguistic processing. Soh *et al.* (1978) studied 13 aphasic patients with left-hemisphere pathologies. When these patients were asked to speak there was a characteristic activation of the frontal lobes, well known for their role in planning and strategic activities, which suggests that the patients were trying to find some way of expressing themselves despite damage to the classical speech areas.

If such techniques were more readily available to brain-function therapists there would be a unique opportunity to evaluate the success of directed stimulation to specific brain regions as simultaneous physiological and behavioural activation.

2 Language and neurophysiological coding

In recent years neuroscientists have begun to pay attention to the contribution made by subcortical structures to linguistic processing. Ojemann (1975) has reviewed the evidence for thalamic involvement in language performance and has concluded that deficits in object-naming can be demonstrated when the left side of the thalamus is involved but not with the right. This asymmetry of function at subcortical levels deserves closer scrutiny as it may hold the key to certain cases of expressive aphasia.

Further technological advances have led to even more intriguing studies of the role of subcortical structures in language processing. Bechtereva, Bundzen, Gogolitsin, Malyshev and Perepelkin (1979) describe a new procedure which may offer a further window on the neurophysiological mechanisms of language and consciousness. Using chronically implanted microelectrodes in patients undergoing surgery for the relief of epilepsy and dyskinesias it was possible to record neuronal firing rates in different subcortical populations. By making recordings of this activity during the perception, retention and production of speech it was possible to scan the resulting record (using computer-automated searches) for specific patterns of firing associated with the verbal stimuli. In this way the authors identified a number of neurophysiological 'codes' representing discrete words. This series of investigations has not been able to identify any 'universal grammar' of neuronal codes—each individual patient produces unique firing patterns for the same stimulus word. However, having established the relevant codes of words for a specific individual it is possible to plot the occurrence of these codes in different subcortical regions.

Bechtereva *et al.* identified a number of distinct phenomena using this methodology including the establishment of informational links in these subcortical systems. The implication of this work points to another threshold of direct observation of the process of consciousness. A further step has been taken towards the solution of the enigma of mind-body relationship.

3 The mind-body question

For centuries scientists, philosophers and religions have debated the relationship between mental experience (consciousness) and the physical body (neurophysiological activity). Some have argued for a distinct separation between the two entities (dualists), others have gathered evidence for the position that neural events give rise to conscious experience (scientific materialists). For at least a century this latter view has dominated both medical and neuropsychological thought and is well portrayed by the writings of Armstrong (1976). Recently however the pioneer of split-brain research, Sperry (1965; 1979), has advanced a view of brain function and consciousness which overturns the conventional position on the mind-body relationship. In the mid-1960s Sperry suggested that it might be possible for mental activity to exert a causal influence on the actual neurophysiological processes taking place in the brain. Rather than consciousness being some by-product of neurophysiological functioning he suggested that mental experience is neither identical with, or reducible to neural events. Nor is Sperry now alone in advancing this thesis; the eminent philosopher of science, Sir Karl Popper, and the equally celebrated neuroscientist, Sir John Eccles, have collaborated on formulating a similar theoretical position (Popper and Eccles 1977) where mental experience (consciousness) exerts a causal influence on neurochemistry and neurophysiology.

These new formulations of the mind-body relationship have profound implications for psychiatry, psychology and neuropsychology in particular. The idea that mind moves matter in the brain brings back long-lost credibility to phenomenological (introspective) methods of study in psychology as well as offering a new impetus to psychophysiological research. Although the notion that specific frames of mind could lead to disruption of somatic processes has a long history in psychology and medicine it is only in recent years that coherent models of these relationships have emerged. Seligman (1975) has introduced the concept of 'learned helplessness' as an explanatory construct to account for diverse mind-body phenomena from depression to the survival of terminal illness.

Although this line of reasoning may well hold the key to future developments in preventative medicine it has immediate implications for the care of the brain-damaged person. Sperry's views could stimulate a new emphasis on the phenomenological investigation of aphasic patients in order to boost motivation, quell emotional distress and inculcate an individual problem-solving approach to recovery of function. It is a truism that motivational state is the *sine qua non* of new learning; the humiliation of brain damage presents an additional emotional burden as well as specific cognitive impairments. The need to recognize these dimensions of brain damage in any comprehensive approach to rehabilitation will be self-evident to clinicians. By gearing directed stimulation to the needs and interests of the individual patient and ensuring that no repetitive failure experiences attend therapy there will come about a gradual rebuilding of confidence in residual and emergent abilities.

Many of the features of this approach to neuropsychological therapy can be seen in the work of Basso, Capitani and Vignolo (1979) who advocate structured stimulation to facilitate a shift from automatic to voluntary responses. Initially this shift is achieved by providing additional saliency in treatment tasks through the use of enriched cues to simulate spontaneous production. As progress occurs these cues are gradually faded out. The authors contend:

> this passage from more automatic to more voluntary constitutes the core of rehabilitation. It consists of a dynamic therapist-patient interplay, which must be carried out with a rapid, pressing rhythm within each single exercise, that is, within a few minutes time. The choice of facilitations and the degree of fading out are not pre-programmed but are intuitively decided at the moment on the basis of the patient's preceding responses. Such continuously renewed attempts to shift upward to a more intentional use of language, if successful, powerfully enhances the patient's motivation. In contrast the repetitive administration of facilitating stimuli is merely a useless and depressing simulation of therapy. Since the aim of rehabilitation is to restore verbal behaviour that can be used in real communication, stimuli and response involve sentences and meaningful words while the use of isolated syllables or phonemes is avoided whenever possible. Special techniques of facilitation, such as melodic intonation or deblocking are employed when indicated (p. 192).

These authors describe the need to enhance saliency during therapy and provide an enriched source of minor-hemisphere cues through the use of spatial markers. In addition this study features individual instruction programmes which acknowledge the importance of patient motivation for outcome. The entire study concerns outcome evaluation in 162 aphasics treated along these lines with an untreated control group of 119 patients. Despite having a major methodological flaw in the allocation of patients to treatment and control groups, it would seem some evidence supports the conclusion that this approach to rehabilitation was very effective, even in cases of longstanding deficit, and was not dependent on clinical subtype of aphasia. Provision of treatment details is relatively rare in neuropsychological therapy yet as Prins, Snow and Wagenaar (1978) point out, rather than ask 'Does therapy contribute to recovery from aphasia?' we should be asking 'What kind of therapy is effective for what type of patient and when, how often, and for how long should it be given to maintain maximum effectiveness?' (p. 193).

Conclusion

Contemporary neuropsychology is in a state of transition; the preoccupations of the past with assessment and cataloguing of dysfunction are gradually being replaced by a vigorous and rigorous concern with rehabilitation. New technology and new conceptions of brain function herald a movement that for too long has been neglected by neuropsychologists. The 1980s may witness a dramatic growth in the numbers of neuropsychologists trained in the skills of investigation and pioneering new approaches to the rehabilitation of brain-injured patients.

4

Hemispheric specialization retraining in aphasia: possibilities and problems

Chris Code

Introduction

A massive literature serves as testimony to the proposition that functional asymmetries for cognitive processing exist between the two hemispheres of the normal brain (Bogen 1969; Gazzaniga 1970; Dimond 1972; Dimond and Beaumont 1974); although the superiority for particular processes appears to be more relative than absolute, and the separate hemispheres are seen by some as performing cognitive tasks in an integrated or cooperative manner (Dimond 1972; Gazzaniga and LeDoux 1978) and by others as operating in competition (Levy 1969). The essential finding of all this research on normal, split-brain and brain-damaged subjects confirms the notion that the left hemisphere in the great majority of right-handers, and most left-handers, possesses a relative superiority for linguistic-analytic cognitive processing, and the right hemisphere is specialized in holistic-Gestalt processing. See Purser (chapter 3) for further discussion. However, recent studies have thrown new light on the linguistic capabilities of the right hemisphere. Zaidel (1976; 1978) has demonstrated that the right hemisphere is capable of the comprehension of language. Butler and Norrsell (1968) and Gazzaniga and associates (Gazzaniga 1977; Gazzaniga, LeDoux and Wilson 1977; Gazzaniga, Volpe, Smylie, Wilson and LeDoux 1979) have provided evidence to show that the right hemisphere may be capable of producing expressive speech. The much studied split-brain subject of the Gazzaniga series of experiments is apparently developing right-hemisphere expressive speech some $3\frac{1}{2}$ years after commissurotomy.

A growing number of studies with normal and aphasic subjects are indicating that the right hemisphere may actually be superior for certain aspects of language; for instance, serial-automatic speech (Larsen, Skinhøj and Lassen 1978), intonation (Blumstein and Cooper 1974) and prosody and affective-emotional language (Ross and Mesulam 1979; Buck and Duffy 1980; Code, 1982).

The *lateral shift hypothesis* holds that, following damage to the left hemisphere, the intact right hemisphere becomes involved in the processing of language to a greater extent than in the normal brain. The hypothesis can be stated at various strengths. A strong version might propose that the right hemisphere is entirely responsible for any recovery following onset, and that increasing improvement is a function of the incremental linguistic abilities of the undamaged side of the brain. A weaker form would postulate that artificial communicative methods that might be successful, owe that success to utilization of intact right-hemisphere cognitive modes (see Rowley, chapter 15, for further discussion). An intermediate and more differential variant might submit that a particular observable characteristic of aphasia is the product of the right hemisphere or of both the undamaged right and the damaged left hemispheres in combination (Nielsen 1946). Coltheart's (1980) model of reading aloud in deep dyslexic patients, for instance, proposes that the left hemisphere processes the expressive speech and the patient makes use of a right-hemisphere orthographic lexicon which is transmitted to the left hemisphere. Errors in reading aloud arise in such patients due to either poor semantic representations or syntactic ability in the right hemisphere, or poor intrahemispheric transmission of semantic information from right to left, depending on the type of error.

The evidence in support of some variant of the lateral shift hypothesis comes from studies using non-invasive neuropsychological techniques for determining lateralization of verbal perception like dichotic listening (Moore and Weidner 1975; Johnson, Sommers and Weidner 1977; Pettit and Noll 1979) and hemi-field viewing (Shai, Goodglass and Barton 1972; Moore and Weidner 1974), and harder neurophysiological evidence using the techniques of carotid barbiturate injection (Kinsbourne 1971; Czopf 1979) and regional cerebral blood flow (Larsen, Skinhøj and Lassen 1978; Skinhøj and Larsen 1980). Strong support comes from cases of recovery from aphasia after left-hemisphere damage, where the patient becomes aphasic a second time following a second lesion, this time to the right hemisphere (Neilson 1946; Searleman 1977); also in cases of left hemispherectomy where patients have been reported to recover language to varying degrees which can only be mediated by the remaining right hemisphere (Smith 1966; Searleman 1977; Zaidel 1978). However, varying degrees of shift may occur in different individual patients, depending on such variables as time-since-onset, age, sex, extent and site of lesion and individual and familial handedness.

Among currently employed therapeutic methods are a number which may encourage right-hemisphere involvement, such as Blissymbolics (Bailey, chapter 16, this volume), melodic intonation therapy (Sparks and Holland 1976) and gestural (Huskins, chapter 11, this volume) and artificial language systems (see Rowley, chapter 15, this volume, for further discussion on this point). Such methods are generally brought in as last resorts when it is clear that recovery of expression will not reach an adequate functional level. Consequently, they are usually tried with the more severe Broca's and global patients. There may be a case for suggesting that such 'right hemisphere' methods might have a more beneficial effect if introduced much earlier into the treatment programme.

The aim of the experiment described in this chapter was to examine the possibilities of encouraging increasing right-hemisphere processing of left-hemisphere linguistic tasks in an aphasic subject. As such, the treatment programmes described were concerned with the perceptual processing of linguistic tasks that the mass of evidence suggests are mediated by the left hemisphere in the normal brain. Therefore, the objective was not to encourage compensatory strategies, but rather to encourage in the undamaged hemisphere the development of those neurocognitive skills for which the right hemisphere appears to be non-specialized. At the same time, the linguistic tasks which made up the programmes were considered to underlie the deficits of the subject of the experiment.

Three experimental programmes were designed to treat via the auditory modality using dichotic listening tapes (Part I), via the visual modality using hemi-field viewing (Part II) and via both modalities using a combined cross-modal (dichotic and hemi-field) programme (Part III). The objectives of the study were, firstly to examine whether such an approach would produce improvement in the subject's communicative abilities as has been suggested (Buffery 1977; Buffery and Burton, 1982); secondly to determine whether the programme would cause any changes in lateral preferences for linguistic material; and thirdly to examine the therapeutic applicability of some experimental techniques and to establish questions for further research. As such, the experiment represents a pilot application and test of neuropsychological theory and methodology.

With methods presently available it was decided that a hemispheric specialization retraining (HSR) programme could best be designed for decoding processes, consequently a patient with predominantly comprehension problems would make the most suitable subject. It was necessary that the subject had undergone regular speech therapy for a number of years and had maximized recovery, so that the subject could act as his own control.

Method

Subject

The subject of the experiment (J.W.) was a 37-year-old male Wernicke's aphasic patient who had suffered a thromboembolic CVA some four years before. Computerized tomography confirmed a left temporal lobe lesion. He had received $3\frac{1}{2}$ years of regular speech therapy before discharge and was considered on the basis of assessment and his clinician's judgement to have maximized recovery.

J.W. is a bachelor, was well educated up to 18 years of age (A level standard), and was a Local Government Officer before his stroke. He now works as a gardener and presents as a well adjusted individual, being very cooperative and well motivated. He is dominantly right-handed (Oldfield 1971) with no family history of sinistrality.

Neuropsychological assessment

Exhaustive testing was carried out before treatment began, and following each part of the programme, in order to establish a baseline against which to measure change in communicative ability and lateral preference, and to eliminate right-hemisphere damage and sensory loss.

Language tests administered were the Porch Index of Communicative Ability (Porch 1971), the Boston Diagnostic Aphasia Examination (Goodglass and Kaplan 1972), the Revised Token Test (De Renzi and Faglioni 1978) the Reporter's Test (De Renzi and Ferrari 1978) and a separate Digit Span Test (Albert and Bear 1974).

The tests of lateral preference for linguistic material were a dichotic CVC word test (Code 1981), a dichotic digit test, a bilateral tachistoscopic CVC word test and single-letter test and a unilateral haptic (tactile) CVC word test and letter test.

Tests carried out to rule out right-hemisphere damage and agnosias included tests for visual, auditory and tactile agnosia, block construction and stick tests and tests of drawing. Investigation of tactile sensation was also carried out. No signs of right-hemisphere damage, agnosia or tactile sensory abnormality were observed. J.W.'s performance on the Coloured Progressive Matrices (Raven 1938a) was also within normal limits, indicating a relatively intact non-verbal intelligence level.

Treatment programme

Assessment revealed that J.W.'s problems lay primarily in comprehension. Comprehension deficit in aphasia is not fully understood although there are some clues as to its nature. An impairment of phonemic discrimination is considered by some to be fundamental (Luria 1970), although empirical support for this view is hard to find (Blumstein, Baker and Goodglass 1977). However, there is evidence which indicates that the ability to analyse rapidly changing formant transitions—a property of the left hemisphere—underlies comprehension deficit (Tallal and Newcombe 1978). Albert and Bear (1974) have shown that the temporal aspects of speech perception are essentially implicated in comprehension loss, such that the patient requires more *time* to understand, and recent dichotic studies provide support for the hypothesis that the left hemisphere is specialized for temporal processing in the normal brain (Mills and Rollman 1979; 1980). In addition, a number of studies have demonstrated that semantic impairment is a factor in comprehension loss (Boller, Kim and Mack 1977).

Current knowledge would therefore suggest that phonemic discrimination, auditory verbal retention and semantic discrimination may be the important factors in auditory comprehension and that an improved right-hemisphere ability in these aspects of language comprehensions should produce positive changes in communicative abilities for J.W.

Part I. In Part I phonemic discrimination and verbal auditory retention deficit were treated using specially constructed dichotic tapes. The phonemic discrimination sub-programme was prepared from a dichotic tape of synthetic stops plus /a/ CV syllables. Discrimination of phonemes by *voice, place* and *voice plus place* was treated by presentation of a syllable to one ear with the simultaneous presentation of another syllable, with the initial stop differing in either voice, place or voice plus place, to the other ear. J.W. was required to verbally report the syllable he heard at his *left* ear (right hemisphere). All stimulus pairs were preceded on the tape by a binaurally presented two-second-long environmental sound in an attempt to 'prime' the right hemisphere. J.W. was required to first report the sound or point to one of an array of six pictures depicting the six sounds used before reporting the left-ear syllable.

A dichotic digit tape was constructed to treat the verbal auditory retention deficit, where two increasing to three pairs of digits were presented with pauses varying between 3 and 1.5 seconds between pairs. For instance, the final set of digits prepared presented three digits to one ear and three digits to the other with a pause of 1.5 seconds between each pair. J.W. had to report as many of the left-ear digits as he could.

Finally in Part I, phonemic discrimination and auditory retention were combined using minimally paired word combinations such as 'bat – pat'. Two increasing to three pairs of words were presented, with 3 decreasing to 2 seconds between pairs. Again, the subject had to report the two or three words he heard at his left ear.

Part II. Part II utilized the tachistoscopic hemifield viewing method to present visual-verbal material to the right hemisphere via the left visual-field (LVF). The tasks involved were letter, digit and CVC word identification and semantic discrimination of words using a three-word odd-one-out task.

Briefly, the method adopted here required the subject to fixate a central small black spot exposed for 1 second. When the spot disappeared, a larger geometric shape (a 1 cm. triangle, square, circle, etc.) was exposed in the central position with the verbal material in the subject's LVF. In order to ensure that material is only seen by the field to which it is directed, it is necessary for exposure to be very brief, with a correct report of the central fixation stimulus. Exposure times were all below 150 ms. throughout the programme. Geometric shapes were used as fixation, again in an attempt to prime the right hemisphere (Kershner, Thomae and Callaway 1977).

Letter naming started with one and increased to three letters with exposure times gradually decreasing from 150 to 100 ms. Digit naming started with three increasing to four digits with exposure ranging from 120 to 80 ms. Single-word naming started with 150 and gradually decreased to 60 ms., and identification of two words ranged from 100 decreasing to 80 ms. The two-word task was made phonologically more difficult and interesting by presenting two words that could be phonologically fused, such as sun – pun (*spun*) and kin – sin (*skin*). J.W. was expected to report both words and also to deduce the fused word.

The odd-one-out semantic discrimination task involved presentation of three CVC words in the LVF at 150 ms. For success, J.W. had to identify and retain all three words in order to be able to state which one was semantically unrelated to the other two. Examples of word triplets used are, hat – bed – tie, gun – cup – pan, car – bus – pig.

Part III. The cross-modal capabilities of dichotic listening and hemi-field viewing were exploited in Part III, by presenting material simultaneously to the right hemisphere via the auditory and visual modalities. Verbal auditory retention and phonemic discrimination were combined, and a same/different paradigm employed. One cross-modal treatment task employed digits and another minimally paired words. In the first sub-programme, two pairs of digits were presented dichotically via tape (two digits to each ear), with a pause of 1.5 seconds between each pair. At the presentation of the first digit pair a central fixation spot was exposed for 1 second on the tachistoscope and on presentation of the second dichotic pair two digits appeared in the LVF with a geometric shape at fixation. Both the tachistoscopic and dichotic digits at the left ear were either identical (same) or both digits in the LVF were different to the dichotically presented digits (different). J.W. was required to report both the fixation shape and say either 'same' or 'different'. Following this sub-programme the task was made more difficult by increasing the number of digits to three at the left ear and three in the LVF exposed for 80 ms.

A task was prepared where one of the three tachistoscopically presented digits was the same as one of the three dichotically presented digits for a 'different' response, or all three visual matched the three auditory digits for a 'same' response. A more difficult further subtask was prepared where two of the three visual digits were the same as the dichotic digits for a 'different' response. Phonemic discrimination was combined with verbal auditory retention by presenting dichotic pairs of minimally paired words simultaneously with words in the subject's LVF for a same/different response.

All stimuli used throughout the HSR programme were presented in sets of 10 and responses recorded on Base 10 response forms (LaPointe 1977). J.W. was seen on a twice-weekly basis in sessions lasting about 40 minutes. This was done in order to avoid any possibility of intensive attention influencing final results. The entire HSR programme covered a period of 19 months with each of the three parts covering approximately the same $6\frac{1}{2}$-months.

Results

Record of treatment

A record of the subject's responses to all three parts of the HSR programme is presented in Figures 4.1 to 4.3. Figure 4.1 shows Base 10 records of progress on Part I, Figure 4.2 shows the record of progress on Part II and Figure 4.3 shows progress on Part III.

A number of points are worth making with regard to J.W.'s ongoing performance during treatment in Part I. There is a great deal of variability of response from one Base 10 to another, and it can be seen—especially in Figure 4.1B (/k/—/g/ discrimination)—that performance for a given Base 10 can almost be predicted by the level of performance on the previous Base 10. This may be a reflection at the intermittent nature of the subject's auditory imperception.

Progress with digit retention (Figures 4.1C and 1D) shows that, in the two-digit with 3-second pauses condition, J.W.'s performance at first deteriorated, then consolidated and reached the criterion of 80 per cent after 41 Base 10s (410 individual trials). This contrasts with performance on two digits with 1.5-second pauses, which should have been more difficult, and performance on three digits with 1.5-second pauses where criterion was reached fairly rapidly after 111 trials.

Progress reporting two to three words with 2-second pauses between them is

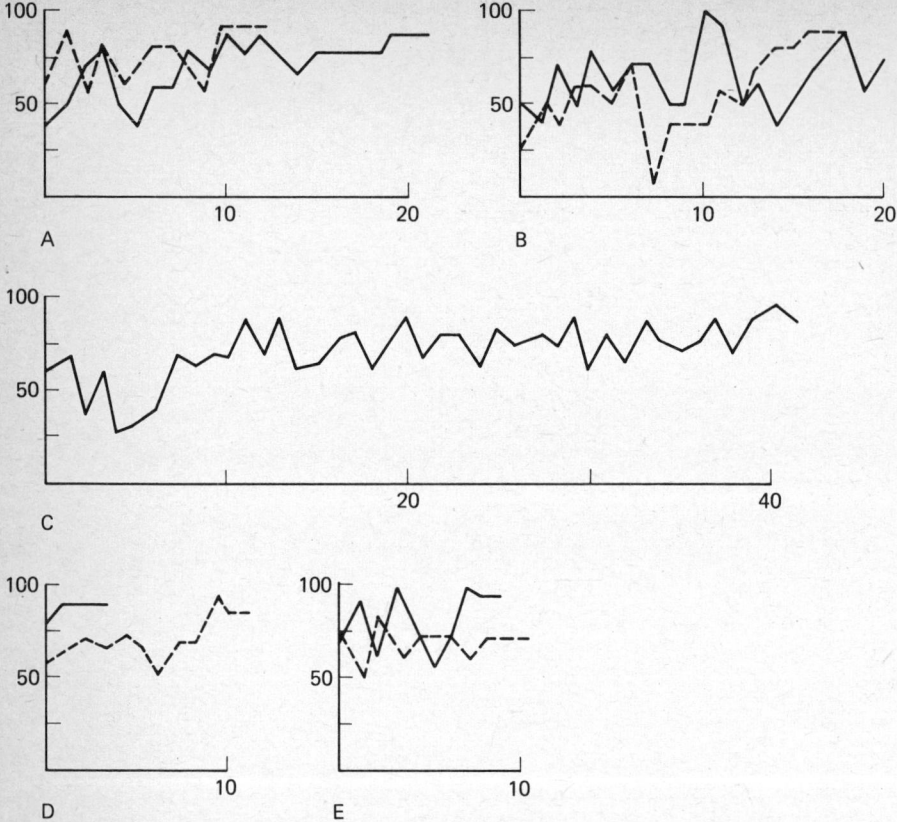

Figure 4.1 Base 10 records of ongoing progress during Part I of the HSR treatment programme. Vertical = percent correct and horizontal = successive Base 10's.
A: solid line—discrimination of initial stops by voice;
   broken line—discrimination of initial stops by place.
B: solid line—discrimination of /k/ and /g/;
   broken line—discrimination of initial stops by voice and place.
C: report of 2 digits at left ear with 3 sec. pause between digits.
D: solid line—report of 2 digits at left ear with 1.5 sec. pause between digits;
   broken line—report of 3 digits at left ear with 1.5 sec. pause between digits.
E: solid line—report of 2 words at left ear with 2 sec. pause between words;
   broken line—report of 3 words at left ear with 3 sec. pause between words.

shown in Figure 4.1E. Progress on two words was erratic but J.W. moved from a baseline of 70 per cent correct to the criterion of 90 per cent in 9 Base 10s. On three words little improvement is seen, despite starting with a high 70 per cent baseline.

Ongoing performance on Part II is shown in Figure 4.2. Improvement from baseline was rapid for three digits, but did not reach criterion for four digits at 100 ms. Single words (Figure 4.2C) shows swift improvement at 150 ms. and 100 ms. and slower progress at 80 ms., but reaching criterion in 110 trials.

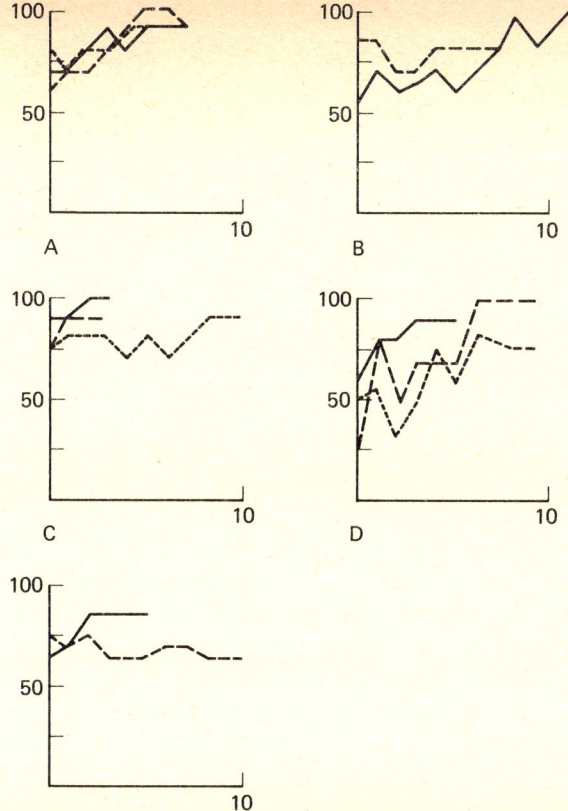

Figure 4.2 Base 10 records of ongoing progress during Part II of the HSR treatment programme. Vertical = percent correct and horizontal = successive Base 10's.
A: solid line—report of single letters at 150 msecs. exposure time;
   wide broken line—report of single letters of 100 msecs. exposure time;
   narrow broken line—report of single letters at 80 msecs. exposure time.
B: solid line—report of 2 letters at 150 msecs. exposure time;
   broken line—report of 3 letters at 150 msecs. exposure time.
C: solid line—report of single words at 150 msecs. exposure time;
   wide broken line—report of single words at 100 msecs. exposure time;
   narrow broken line—report of single words at 70 msecs. exposure time.
D: solid line—report of 2 CVC words at 150 msecs. exposure time;
   wide broken line—phonological fusion of 2 words to produce one 's' blend word;
   narrow broken line—semantic discrimination of 1 odd man out of 3 CVC words.
E: solid line—report of 3 digits of 100 msecs. exposure time;
   broken line—report of 4 digits at 100 msecs. exposure time.

Processing of two and three words under different conditions showed good progress at 50 ms. The phonological fusion task (processing of two words at 100 ms.) started with a baseline of 40 per cent and climbed erratically to 100 per cent in 90 trials, and the three-word odd-one-out semantic discrimination task reached the 80 per cent criterion in 100 trials. Reporting single letters at three different exposure times showed steady improvement in scores, as did reporting two and three letters at 150 ms.

Figure 4.3 presents the Base 10 records of Part III of the HSR programme. Progress on two digits at exposure times of 80 and 100 ms. was rapid, and treatment soon moved on to the three-digit conditions. Progress was good where one digit at the left ear and in the LVF were the same, but slower when two digits were the same at the ear as in the LVF at 80 ms.

The record of progress for cross-modal same/different responses for words

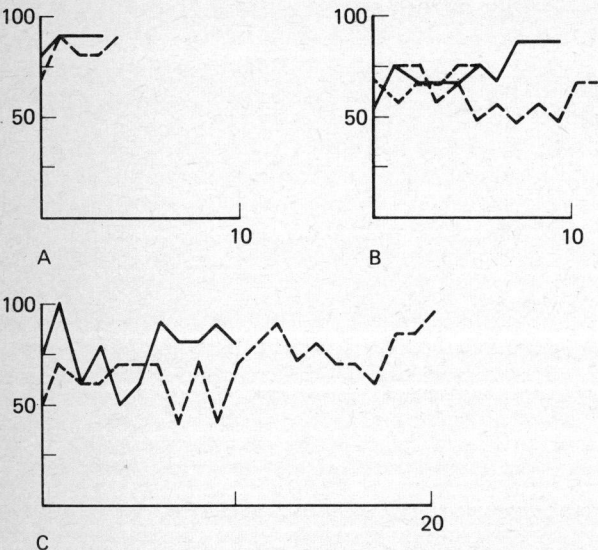

Figure 4.3 Base 10 records of ongoing progress during Part III of the HSR treatment programme. Vertical = percent correct and horizontal = successive Base 10's.

A: solid line—same/different discrimination of 2 digits at 100 msecs. exposure time; broken line—same/different discrimination of 2 digits at 80 msecs. exposure time.

B: narrow broken line—same/different discrimination of 2 digits at 100 msecs. with 2 digits in LVF and LE the same;
wide broken line—same/different discrimination of 3 digits at 80 msecs. exposure with 2 digits in LVF and LE the same;
solid line—same/different discrimination of 3 digits at 80 msecs. exposure with just 1 digit in LVF and LE the same.

C: solid line—same/different discrimination of single dichotic pair of words at 150 msecs. exposure time;
broken line—same/different discrimination of double dichotic pair of words at 150 msecs. exposure time.

(Figure 4.3C) shows that erratic progress was made for single and double words where criterion was reached in both conditions.

Language tests

J.W.'s scores on a range of language tests administered pre-treatment and following Parts I, II and III are presented in Tables 4.1 to 4.3 and Figures 4.4 to 4.6.

PICA Modality Response Summaries for gestural and verbal subtests are shown in Figure 4.4 and gestural and verbal means in Table 4.1. Firstly, it is of interest to note that the pre-treatment scores on the PICA show that J.W. had made a good recovery in a number of subtest areas. According to the High—Low Gap analysis which is possible with the PICA (Porch 1967), J.W. had maximized his recovery. A large discrepancy would indicate that there is much recovery that can be made

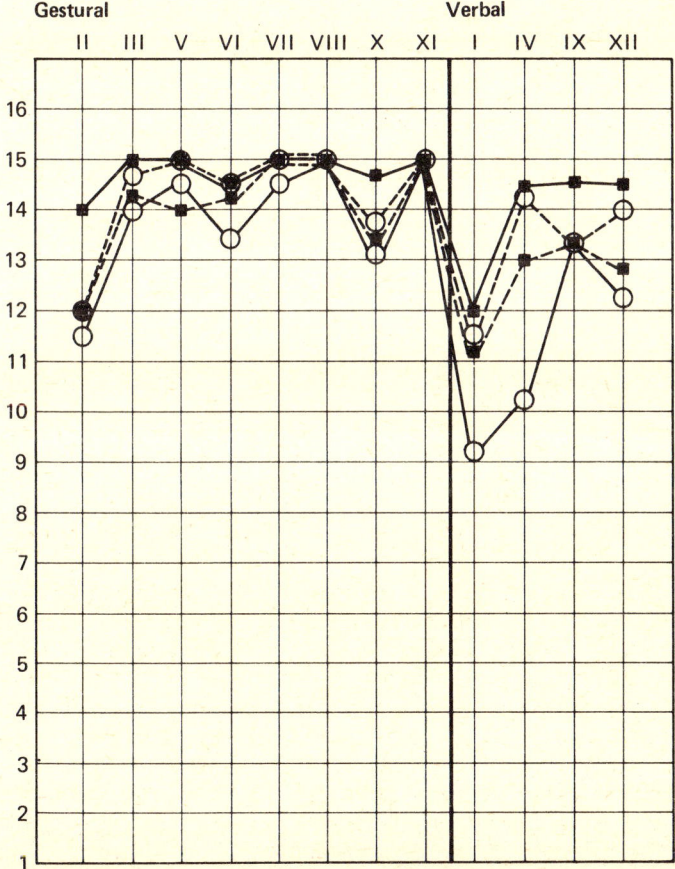

Figure 4.4 PICA Modality Response Summary for gestural and verbal subtests at pre-treatment (0———0), post-Part I (■-----■), post-Part II (0-----0) and post-Part III (■———■).

Table 4.1 Pre- and post-test PICA gestural and verbal means compared to test-retest data from Porch (1967)

	Pre-test	Post-part I	change	Post-part II	change	Post-part III	change	Overall change	Test-retest differences
Gestual means	14·00	14·12	+0·12	14·38	+0·26	14·87	+0·49	+0·87	0·30
Verbal means	11·30	12·50	+1·20	13·47	+0·97	13·97	+0·5	+2·67	0·44

while a low or non-existent gap indicates that the patient is unlikely to make further improvement. J.W.'s scores produced no high—low gap indicating that further progress was unlikely.

Of further interest in Figure 4.4 and Table 4.1 is that improvement was made in the subtests which were most depressed, with most progress in verbal subtests. Steady positive change can be seen throughout the treatment programme. Also shown in Table 4.1 is a comparison of changes in gestural and verbal means with the test-retest differences on the PICA reported by Porch (1967). The subtest scores of each administration of the PICA were also subjected to matched pairs t test analysis, although it should be noted that there are arguments against applying statistical analysis to single-case designs (Hersen and Barlow 1976). A comparison of scores with test-retest differences may therefore make more clinical sense, where positive changes in scores which are higher than the test-retest differences can be considered to be significant changes. The test-retest difference for the gestural mean reported by Porch is 0.30 and Table 4.1 shows that this figure is exceeded only after the cross-modal sub-programme, as well as for the overall change between the pre-treatment test and the final test. However, changes in the verbal means following each part of the HSR programme are all higher than the test-retest figures. Matched pairs t test were applied to the subtest scores following each administration of the PICA, and comparison of pre-treatment and post-Part I scores produced a significant result ($t = 2.916$; $p < .01$). A similar analysis of post-Part I and post-Part II scores produced a significant result ($t = 2.766$; $p < .01$), and comparison of post-Part II and post-Part III scores was also significant, but less so ($t = 2.253$; $p < .025$; $df = 11$). These results would indicate modest but significant improvement in general communicative ability throughout the HSR programme.

J.W.'s scores on the revised Token Test show an initially severe comprehension deficit on pre-test (Table 4.2), which shows modest change by the HSR programme especially the final post-treatment administration of the test. The scores were subjected to matched pairs t test analysis following each administration of the Token Test, with the result that comparison of pre-treatment and post-Part I did not reach significance; comparison of post-Part II with post-Part III was insignificant ($t = 1.964$; $p < .10$; $df = 5$) and a comparison of the pre-treatment and final Token Test scores was significant at the .025 level ($t = 2.803$; one tailed test; $df = 5$). The Reporter's Test is De Renzi and Ferrari's (1978) high level expressive version of the revised Token Test (Table 4.3). It assesses the patient's ability to report the Token Test actions of the tester to a fictitious third person. The test was administered primarily as an objective evaluation of J.W.'s verbal formulation and rate of utterance pre- and post-treatment. J.W. made few syntactic or anomic errors. Figure 4.5 shows a large increase in verbal formulation errors coupled with a reduction in rate of utterance following Part I of the treatment programme. The number of formulation errors made during the test reduced to 8 following Part II and Part III, but the rate of utterance remained high until the final assessment following Part III. A comparison of pre-treatment and final post-treatment rate of utterances and formulation errors shows that while the former remained almost identical the latter were reduced by half.

Table 4.2 Pre- and Post-Test Token Test scores and classification

	Pre-Test	Post-Part I	Post-Part II	Post-Part III	Overall change
Score (Max. Score = 36)	11	14	12	16.5	5.5
(% correct)	(30·5%)	(38·8%)	(33·3%)	(45·8%)	(15·3%)
Classification	Severe	Severe	Severe	Severe/Moderate	
(Severe range = 9–16)					

Table 4.3 Assessment of verbal fluency on the Reporter's Test

	Pre-Test	Post-Part I	Post-Part II	Post-Part III
Overall time to respond	2 mins. $49\frac{1}{2}$ secs.	3 mins. $34\frac{1}{2}$ secs.	3 mins. 23 secs.	2 mins. $48\frac{1}{2}$ secs.
Mean time per response	8·04 secs.	10·1 secs.	9·6 secs.	8 secs.
Number of verbal formulation errors	19	31	8	8

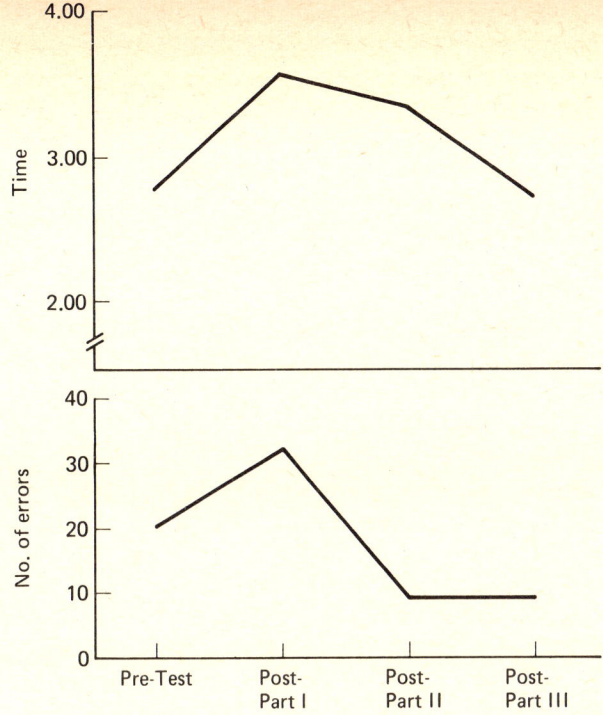

Figure 4.5 Pre- and post-test performances on the Reporter's Test. The top graph shows rate of utterance (the time taken to complete the required verbal responses) and the bottom graph shows the number of verbal formulation errors produced at each test time.

Figure 4.6 presents J.W.'s performance on auditory retention of three digits under three conditions. Ten trigrams of digits were presented in each condition, making 30 digits in all. In the first condition, three digits were presented with pauses of 5 seconds between digits; in the second with 3 seconds between digits; and in the third with 0.5 seconds between digits. This test is based on Albert and Bear (1974) who found that the more time patients were given to comprehend material, the more was retained. The upper part of Figure 4.6 shows overall number of digits retained under each condition at each test administration, and the lower part, the number of complete trigrams (all three digits) retained. Improvement under all three conditions can be noted with the most dramatic change following Part I of the HSR programme. There is a small deterioration in performance following Part III.

Tests of lateral preference

It will be recalled that the six tests employed to measure lateral preferences for linguistic material were a dichotic word and dichotic digit test, a tachistoscopic word and letter test and a haptic word and letter test. Figure 4.7 presents a breakdown of these tests which were administered pre-treatment and following each part

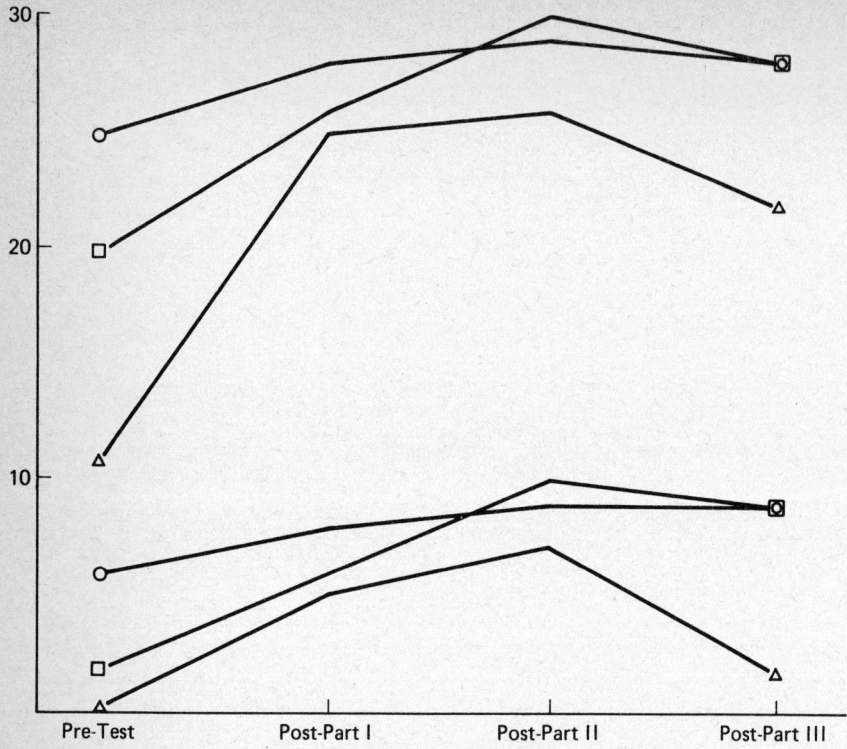

Figure 4.6 Pre- and post-test performances on auditory retention of 3 digits at three presentation rates: with a 5 second pause between digits (0———0), a 3 second pause between digits (□———□) and a 0.5 second pause between digits (△———△). The top part of the graph shows overall number of digits retained at each presentation rate, and the lower part of the graph the number of complete trigrams retained at each rate.

of the HSR programme. Initial testing shows a left ear, eye and hand preference on all tests suggesting shift to the right hemisphere for linguistic perception. Following Part I there is an increase in left preference in all but the tachistoscopic word test which shows a reversal back to right visual field preference. As the latter result is in gross disagreement with the other measures, and left preference was observed to increase throughout the programme, it might be considered to be an artifact. Following the initial increase in left preference, and ignoring the apparent artifact, it can be observed that the increase was maintained throughout the programme, producing a complete right-ear extinction in the case of the dichotic material by the end of Part II. The haptic tests, however, do not show an increasing left-hand preference, but remain fairly stable.

Conclusions and discussion

The subject of this experiment was a Wernicke's aphasic patient four years post-

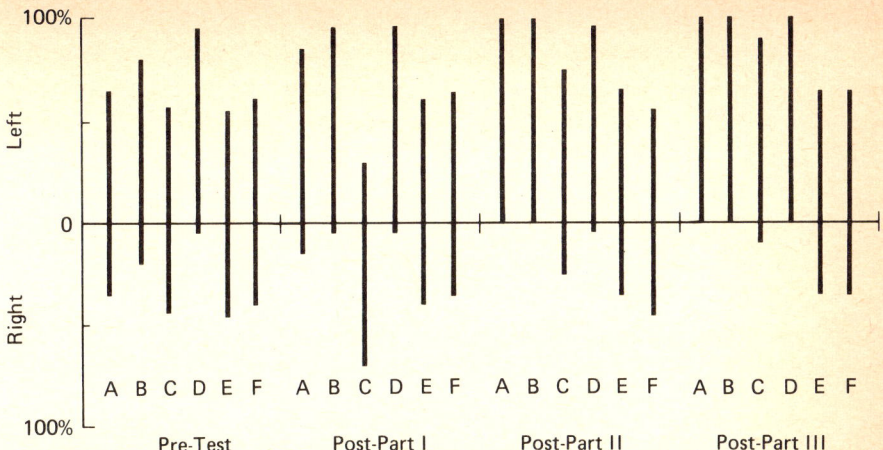

Figure 4.7 Pre-treatment and post-treatment performance on a range of tests of lateral preference for verbal material. (A) dichotic CVC word test; (B) dichotic digit test; (C) tachistoscopic CVC word test; (D) tachistoscopic single letter test; (E) unilateral haptic CVC word test; (F) unilateral haptic single letter test. Scores are expressed in terms of percentage of left and right preference.

onset who had made a maximum recovery and was acting as his own control. He underwent an hemispheric specialization retraining programme using a dichotic listening and hemi-field viewing paradigm aimed at improving the propositional linguistic processing capacity of his intact right hemisphere, especially in comprehension ability which constituted his main deficit area. Gradual improvement was recorded from session to session on treatment tasks, significant improvement was observed in testing of general communicative ability (PICA), modest change in testing non-redundant comprehension of language (Token Test), modest change in verbal fluency (Reporter's Test) and dramatic positive change was noted in auditory retention of digits. Pre-treatment lateral preference tests revealed a dominant left-ear, left visual-field and left-hand preference for linguistic material providing grounds to suppose that the subject had made a shift to the undamaged right hemisphere for linguistic perception before treatment began. Left-ear and left visual-field preferences increased markedly following treatment, with the exception of a tachistoscopic word test following Part I which produced a right visual-field preference. This was taken to be an artifact. On a linguistic haptic test left-hand response-times increased following Part I, but remained stable throughout the rest of the programme.

In most respects the experiment described should be seen as a pilot study which had identified more possibilities and problems than it has provided answers. Any conclusions, therefore, must be tentative. However, a number of points can be made with regard to the results.

Assuming that the treatment material is arriving at the right hemisphere, there is clearly no guarantee that it is not transferring over to the left hemisphere for processing. At first sight the obvious control would be to note reaction times during treatment and to discard any response above what might be considered the inter-hemispheric transfer time. There are a number of problems with this approach, however. Firstly, there is little agreement about the time it takes for information to cross from one hemisphere to the other. Cohen (1977) observes that a variety of experiments have suggested that inter-hemispheric transfer.time ranges from 4 m.sec. to 60 m.sec., and that the size of the difference probably varies between trials, between tasks and between subjects. Moreover, the aphasic patient who can responed to a verbal task at less than 60 m.sec. probably does not exist. Future experiments in this area might consider using EEG or regional cerebral blood flow to determine whether there is left-hemisphere involvement during treatment, although it is by no means certain that these technically complex techniques are at a level of development where they can answer such questions (Dr W.C. McCallum and Dr Stuart Butler, personal communications).

The variability between and within language test scores throughout the treatment programme highlights the necessity of using tighter designs in such single-case studies. The results provide some support for the view that general communicative competence improved as a consequence of the HSR programme. The results of the digit-retention test would suggest that there was dramatic improvement in a specific skill thought to underlie comprehension, which appears to be reflected in the Token Test results which showed modest positive change. At the same time, objective measurement of verbal fluency showed modest improvement at the end of treatment.

The importance of using an extensive laterality battery is demonstrated by the subject's apparent reversal of visual-field preference on one test following Part I and increasing RVF preference on the other hemi-field test. The results of these tests show that although there was a gradual increase in left-ear and LVF preference throughout treatment, no claims should be made for increased right-hemisphere processing of verbal perceptual material. After Part II of the programme both the auditory and visual modalities must be considered contaminated insofar as the increases in left-ear and visual-field preferences are possibly a function of the treatment *methods* and not a true indication of *hemispheric preference*. The subject had a great deal of exposure to the dichotic and tachistoscopic procedures and this would presumably be sufficient in itself to produce increased left-ear and visual-field scores. J.W. showed a significant left-hand preference for verbal material on pre-test, and the haptic tests were used as control lateral preference tests—the tactile modality being uncontaminated by the treatment methods. The left-hand preference was maintained throughout treatment but did not increase, and an increase would have been necessary to support any claim for additional right-hemisphere involvement in linguistic processing following the HSR programme. It should be noted, however, that despite the mass of literature on ear and visual-field asymmetrics, evidence for asymmetry in haptic processing of linguistic material is less abundant, although it is available (Oscar-Berman, Rehbein, Porfert and Goodglass 1978). This is perhaps partly because tactile linguistic material can also be regarded visuospatially, and consequently processed predominantly by the right hemisphere, and partly because the tactile modality does not function normally as a perceptual channel for propositional language.

In some respects the choice of subject for this study constitutes a very stringent test of an HSR hypothesis, as J.W. had made a very good functional recovery, despite a severe comprehension deficit on the Token Test. His initially good PICA results would indicate that he was able to adopt a number of compensatory strategies to overcome comprehension difficulties. It is a matter for speculation as to whether a similar subject might show more eventual recovery of comprehension if treated with an HSR approach much earlier post-onset, during the so-called period of spontaneous recovery.

Future studies might consider more severe patients as experimental subjects as well as different clinical types of aphasic patients. Different materials and modality combinations might be used, perhaps leaving the visual or auditory modality uncontaminated so that it can be used as a control modality. A promising aspect of the experiment was the subject's positive response to the digit-retention dichotic task and this would appear to warrant further investigation, perhaps comparing the progress of two well matched groups to a dichotic and non-dichotic treatment regime.

A positive outcome of this study is that hitherto purely experimental techniques may be adapted for treatment purposes, and fairly conventional treatment material can be channelled more directly to undamaged areas using these methods. In this way, the possibly inhibiting influence of the damaged left hemisphere might be bypassed. Many variations are possible: for instance, short comprehension passages might be recorded on separate channels of a stereo tape recorder and the patient asked to attend to the left-ear passage. Performance might then be compared to the patient's non-dichotic responses. Inexpensive tape-slide self-instructional machines might be easily adapted to present visual and auditory material directly to the right hemisphere for reading or naming tasks, or for teaching an artificial language which utilizes intact right-hemisphere cognitive modes.

The results of this experiment are sufficiently encouraging to justify further investigation; but in order that such approaches be stringently tested, a variety of studies using different carefully controlled designs seems to be desirable.

Acknowledgements The author is grateful to W.A. Lishman and Christopher Colbourne for the synthetic dichotic syllable tape used as treatment material in this experiment; to Helen Wynne and Eirion Jones for help in locating the subject and to J.W. himself for his patience, cooperation and good humour. A special acknowledgement is due to the late Stuart Dimond for his support, criticisms and time.

Linguistic Perspectives

Linguistics has played a significant role in advancing our understanding of aphasia in recent years. The discipline provides a descriptive framework for the classification of aphasic language and theoretical models which can help to guide remediation. In this section Hatfield and Shewell present therapeutic methods based on a linguistic description, and Patterson, Purell and Morton's psycholinguistic experiment examines 'phonemic cueing' for the facilitation of word-finding, a traditional technique which is widely used in aphasia therapy. Hatfield and Shewell emphasize the need for therapy to be theoretically based and Patterson et al.'s study highlights the requirement that therapeutic methods should be subjected to careful empirical examination.

5

Some applications of linguistics to aphasia therapy

Frances M. Hatfield and Christina Shewell

Introduction: the need for a linguistic basis in aphasia therapy

This chapter examines the need to apply some of the insights of modern linguistic science to the remediation of aphasia and offers a few concrete suggestions of therapeutic techniques intended to fill part of this need. The approach described is therefore a practical one, and the goals realistic. Nevertheless, whatever the limitations of staff and facilities, the explicit concern of anyone working with aphasic patients must be to lead each patient to a fuller use of language and thereby to richer personal and social activity. Implicit in this goal is the endeavour to understand the nature of language itself and to be in a position to devise scientifically based rehabilitation.

Although any concept of language includes both production and reception this chapter has to be selective, focusing mainly on production. Our general orientation to aphasia therapy is stated and some examples of our techniques are given. These may contribute usefully to the direct work on language that will surely be an important component of the total therapeutic plan for all but the most confused and deteriorated aphasic patients. Concentration on linguistics—in particular, that branch called Structural Linguistics—is not intended to imply a primacy of this discipline in its contribution to aphasiology; recognition of the essential role played by other sciences such as neuropsychology and neurology is taken for granted.

Structural Linguistics is that branch of synchronic linguistics which looks at each language as a set of interrelated systems of elements—sounds, words, etc.—which have no validity independent of the relations between them; it contrasts with comparative linguistics (or comparative philology), historical linguistics and other branches. The realization that language is hierarchically organized and rule-governed allows the disordered language of both adult and child patients to be described in an exhaustive, consistent and economic way. A thorough grounding in phonetics has long been established as a *sine qûa non* for speech therapists; it is necessary to identify with precision what is wrong with each patient's sound system, and for that an understanding of the phonemic system of the normal speaker of the language is essential. As Trim (1963 p. 35) has noted, 'a malfunction can be evaluated only when set against normal function'. However, it took much longer for the same status to be accorded to all the other branches of linguistics.

The linguist who influenced these therapists most strongly was almost certainly Jakobson, through his publication with Halle of *Fundamentals of Language* in 1956, and somewhat later through his contribution to the seminal CIBA symposium on language disorders (Jakobson 1964). Jakobson elaborated his own theory of language breakdown in aphasia and also sought to apply his interpretations to Luria's typology, which had already achieved wide recognition (Jakobson 1964; Jakobson and Halle 1956). Therapists subsequently tried to relate other linguistic theories to their interpretation of aphasic patients' difficulties; for example, transformational generative grammar, as propounded by Harris (1951) and Chomsky (1957, 1965), and some notions of Case grammar (Fillmore 1968) and Structural Semantics (Lyons 1963). A further awareness of ways in which linguistic analysis might be applied to aphasia was encouraged by Trim (1963) and, more recently, by MacMahon (1972) and Crystal, Fletcher and Garman (1976).

In the rest of Europe aphasiologists were rather quicker off the mark in including linguistics in the team approach. Jakobson describes the 1943 Amsterdam meeting of aphasiologists and linguists as one of the first steps towards a joint investigation of language disorders. This meeting was largely inspired by Grewel who was a strong advocate of the need to apply linguistics to aphasiology (1951, 1963). In Paris the linguist Dubois was collaborating with Hécaen throughout the early 1960s (Dubois, Irigaray, Marcie and Hécaen 1967); in West Germany professional linguists were directly concerned with assessment and even treatment of patients in centres such as Bonn and Aachen. And there were other notable partnerships, for example in Poland and East Germany, in particular Weigl and Bierwisch (1970). In Russia Luria had long been linguistically minded. There were also centres in other continents where the participation of linguists in the team was taken for granted.

In spite of the gradual extension of the study of linguistics and its application by aphasia specialists, most linguistic-aphasic papers published in the past 20 years have focused on analysis rather than therapy, as the recent survey by Lesser (1978) demonstrates. But therapy, based on assessment, is the primary aim of the approach described here.

Application of linguistics to the analysis of aphasia before therapy

General principles underlying the aims of assessment and therapy

The firmly held conviction expressed here is that therapy should be throughout *rational* and also *specific* to the form of aphasia. 'Rational' does not simply imply sensible here, when describing therapy, it means that the therapy is based on a well-thought-out theory, whether linguistic or psychological. This contrasts with therapy based on tradition or on intuition unsupported by explicit interpretation of past experience. The word 'specific', when used here, means that therapy is carefully chosen for each particular form of the disorder. The authors reject the notion of a unitary form of aphasia as postulated by Schuell, Jenkins and Jiménez-Pabon (1964); Bay (1964) and some others, but they accept, along with Goodglass and Kaplan of Boston (1972), whose assessment procedure they use, the concept of *qualitatively* distinct patterns of language deficit, with clear implications of the need for different types of remediation. That certain of these specific patterns of language loss correlate approximately with lesions in specific cortical regions is irrelevant to the type of therapy, although relevant to certain kinds of neurophysiological models formulated to account for the deficits. Thus Broca's aphasia is characterized by relative preservation of elementary naming, comprehension and reading aloud, in the context of a breakdown of articulation and fluency, while Wernicke's aphasia has the characteristics of good articulation and fluency, along with impaired comprehension and repetition, and copious paraphasias. Luria's (1970) typology is equally specific as to the underlying defects of each of his six principal forms of aphasia, which roughly fit in with the Boston classification. Moreover, his schemes of therapy are quite distinct for the different forms of aphasia. Both the Boston classification and Luria's lend themselves more readily to linguistic analysis.

In addition to the above recommendations some general principles are described which are not directly concerned with linguistics. For any therapy to be effective, and to be shown to the effective, the assumption is that it must be intensive, at least in the early stages, a precept which it is seldom possible to observe. Finally, the therapist must be selective within his or her case material, exercising discrimination and imagination in shaping the therapeutic approach to the needs of patients with widely differing personalities, ages and states of intellectual and emotional readiness for direct, concentrated treatment even of short duration. Gloning, Trappl, Heiss and Quatember (1976) list 19 variables such as general cognitive deterioration, age and emotional state, that may affect prognosis and these must therefore be taken into account when planning any structured therapy.

Linguistic refinements in assessment: four levels of linguistic analysis

Subtests of greater linguistic refinement need to be grafted on to the Boston assessment to ascertain more precisely which levels or aspects of language are affected and which are comparatively well retained. Using the terms in the Structuralist sense of De Saussure (1916) and others, the most important levels for the linguistic analysis of aphasia are (i) segmental phonology and prosody; (ii) morphology and syntax; (iii) the lexical-semantic (iv) functional aspects of communication for the individual in society.

Breakdown may occur at one level only, e.g. in the lexical-semantic or phonological, or across several levels (Hatfield, 1972). Correlations may be seen between the patterns of breakdown at different levels, and certain clinical types of aphasia. For example, the Broca aphasic has difficulty predominantly in segmental phonology, prosody, syntax and morphology; the Conduction aphasic predominantly in segmental phonology; the Anomic patient at the lexical-semantic level, and the Wernicke's aphasic at the segmental phonological, lexical-semantic and functional (pragmatic) levels of language. Therapy should logically concentrate on improving one aspect, by direct or indirect methods, without neglecting others. Thus work at the phonemic level might progress from reacquisition of single phonemes to combining them in single words and sentences, thereby concurrently introducing practice at the lexical-semantic and syntactic levels.

Illustrations of analysis at different levels

There are various steps in full linguistic analysis. The patient's segmental phonological behaviour has to be assessed in full, using repetition of phonemes, syllables, words and sentences. Phonemic discrimination is also examined.

The prosodic features of intonation, stress, tempo, rhythmicity and pause should be examined, using a transcription of a dialogue between patient and therapist. This dialogue also serves as a basis for the syntactic analysis, where clause, phrase and morphological structure is examined. Further samples of speech may be elicited by leading questions or using story-completion tasks such as those used by Goodglass, Gleason, Bernholtz and Hyde (1972). Here responses may demonstrate that a patient can produce a certain structure for which the evidence was lacking in spontaneous conversation. At the lexical-semantic level, the effects of a number of relevant variables derived from psycholinguistics as well as linguistics can be noted, such as word frequency and concreteness or 'imageability' (Richardson 1976a). It may also be of clinical value to note the proportion of content words to function words in the patient's speech.

Comprehension of connected speech must also be examined to assess the importance of all the above factors for the patient. Some patients fall back on semantic strategies in trying to understand syntactic structures and the examiner will look for evidence of this. Zurif and Caramazza (1976) found that Conduction and Broca aphasic patients utilized semantic strategies to comprehend embedded-clause sentences, resulting in better decoding of non-reversible sentences such as,

> The apple the boy is eating is red.

than reversible sentences such as,

> The boy the girl is chasing is tall.

The use of semantic order strategies in comprehension has been reported by many other researchers, for example, in decoding sentences using the temporal prepositions *before* and *after* (Kotten 1977); comprehending active and passive sentences in direct and 'reversed' order (Akhutina 1978). Syntax and semantics can clearly not be entirely separated in a description of language performance.

The functional aspect of language covers more than the linguistic term pragmatic. It relates to the use of language in varying social contexts, which may be accompanied by various types of non-verbal communication, such as gesture, facial expression, drawings and other 'self-help' devices, all so important for the severely disabled aphasic.

This type of linguistic profile is illustrated by giving two clinical examples. The summary only is presented. The focus here is on productive speech, but the patients had difficulty in other modalities.

(1) Broca-type aphasic. Mr C.H. was a 61-year-old driving-school manager when he sustained a left CVA in 1977. Three months post-onset he showed the following pattern of linguistic deficit:
Segmental Phonology: Severe articulatory dyspraxia limited his phonological

system to a few consonant + vowel combinations. Consonants usually plosives; particular difficulty with fricatives and affricates.
Prosody: Utterances still restricted to single words, therefore prosodic analysis of only certain features was possible. All words produced with the same loud volume, but with preservation of word-stress. He used a range of intonation on these words, in expressing meanings such as assertion, interrogation, doubt, but as the syntactic units were so limited attitudinal meanings were not always clear.
Syntax: One-element utterances only were usually produced.
Lexical-semantic: Limited to a few object names and adjective-type words. Utterances always semantically appropriate at single-word level, although ambiguity often resulted from the incompleteness of the utterance.
Functional communication aspect: Facial expressions, gestures and eye and finger pointing used in an effort to clarify his meaning to the listener. Patient very aware of his difficulties, as comprehension and self-monitoring were fairly good.

(2) **Wernicke-type aphasic.** Mrs N.D. was a 62-year-old retired nursing sister who suffered a left posterior subarachnoid haemorrhage in 1978. Three months later her linguistic profile was very different from Mr C.H.'s.
Segmental Phonology: All English phonemes present in her fluent speech output in spite of frequent phonemic paraphasias both in conversation and repetition tasks.
Prosody: A wide range of intonational patterns in connected speech with fast tempo but frequent short pauses before content words. Intra-word stress well preserved but sentence stress frequently inappropriate to the apparently intended meaning.
Syntax: Complex syntactic structure, with frequent use of lengthy, post-modified clauses which further reduced intelligibility.
Lexical-semantic: Frequent neologisms both in conversation and naming tasks. She was just beginning to be aware of these. Semantic and communicative intention usually difficult to deduce from the speech flow.
Functional communication aspect: Mrs N.D.'s excessive fluency continued in a variety of social contexts. Being unaware of her communication problems due to severe receptive disturbance and self-monitoring defect, she used no non-verbal cues to disambiguate her meaning.

Aphasia therapy with a linguistic basis

Using this approach, therapy aims to help a patient to move from a given state of functioning at one level of language to a higher, more elaborated state. This will also involve other levels of language, using a variety of remedial techniques. These will be modified in accordance with the patient's own interests and explicit wishes, since any therapeutic relationship must fundamentally reflect a collaborative partnership. Wiegel-Crump's (1976) description of an experiment in therapy is a good example of how it is possible to be both structured and imaginative; she used three different syntactic constructions aimed at improving four specific areas of linguistic functioning and showed that structured therapy effected significantly more improvement than general language stimulation.

Selection of linguistic structures on grounds of utility to the patient, and their order of presentation

In selecting linguistic structures for practice it is most important that these should be communicatively useful to the patient and presented in a linguistic hierarchy based on the premise that mastery of one structure may presuppose that of another. The practical utility of a particular structure is crucial to the patient's motivation and, as far as possible, even work at the phonological level should include tasks in a context. To give an example at the syntactic level, where the therapist was aiming at expanding utterances to two-element level, Mr C.H. frequently wanted to talk about himself or his family; therefore practice of Subject-Verb combinations used subjective pronouns and family names extensively as realizations of the grammatical subject, in preference to introducing other variations of the subject which were of less immediate utility to the patient and less frequent in the colloquial language generally. These considerations are often forgotten in therapy. For instance, Naeser (1975) recommends that one syntactic structure to be practised early on, should be the sentence-type *The woman opens the door*. Not only is the present habitual tense far less frequent in normal speech than the present progressive but the substitution of the one for the other alters the meaning. Use of the progressive present tense is preferred for all verbs but the stative ones, such as *feel, see, know*, except when habitual action is directly intended (and then the habitual form would be introduced *after* the progressive).

The question of order of presentation may suggest an inherent order of difficulty of linguistic structures. This is not answered by simply following the order of child language development, or of turning to English-as-a-Foreign-Language procedures. There have already been a few studies of syntactic therapy for different types of aphasic patient (e.g. Grunwell and Davies 1975), which suggest a reasonable order for therapists to follow. Helm (1979) also states that she sees a natural order of complexity for syntax retraining for Broca's aphasics based on a paper by Goodglass, Gleason, Bernholtz and Hyde (1972). In this paper patients' responses in a series of story-completion tasks were examined. However, aphasic patients continually surprise their relatives and therapists by spontaneous utterances of an unexpectedly complex kind and these must be reinforced and included where appropriate in future tasks.

Experiments have also been carried out to establish a rank order of difficulty of comprehension of syntactic structures in aphasia (Parisi and Pizzamiglio 1970; Lesser 1974) and it is possible that this might contribute further to establishing a similar order of difficulty for production—not necessarily the same for each form of aphasia. In addition, there have been studies of phonology and lexicon suggesting a suitable progression of therapeutic tasks (Rochford and Williams 1962; 1963; 1965).

Although at the beginning of this section the authors have dismissed any suggestion of directly following either the presumed order of acquisition of language structures in childhood, or that deemed suitable for foreign language students, they would like to mention that both areas may provide 'teaching' material which can be adapted to the needs of certain patients. Moreover, rejection of an overall conception of aphasia such as Schuell's need not preclude the judicious selection of some of the therapeutic exercises advocated by these writers. The further development of specifically designed therapeutic materials is, however, essential.

Some applications of some theories

It is in the area of relative complexity of syntactic structure that some aspects of early transformational-generative grammar (Chomsky 1965) have been found applicable. With this model, the second of the following two sentences (each of nine words) is more 'complex' than the first:

(i) The rabbit ran quickly round the old gate.
(ii) The rabbit I saw in the garden grew bigger.

According to the theory, Sentence (ii) would be more easily understood by breaking it down as follows:

(iii) I saw the rabbit.
The rabbit was in the garden.
The rabbit grew bigger.

Goodglass, Blumstein, Gleason, Hyde, Green and Statlender (1979) found empirically this to be the case: an embedded sentence was more easily understood by Broca aphasic patients if it was broken down into its constituent two (or three) propositions. This rearrangement made little difference to the Wernicke and Conduction aphasic patients in the experiment.

On the other hand, linguistic theory has also pointed to the close relationship between different sentences of different syntactic types; these relationships have been exploited by Weigl and Bierwisch (1970). These two researchers found that their practice of one sentence-type with an aphasic patient had the effect of deblocking production of other sentences different in their surface structure but all related to the same deep structure; for example, active, declarative sentences and their corresponding passives, interrogative transformations. Both inherent difficulties and anticipated facilitations should be borne in mind when planning therapy for syntax.

There are other models of language structure which can have relevance to therapy and Jakobson's is one. Jakobson stresses the two modes of arrangement for linguistic units—combination and selection—as fundamental to the description of any linguistic sign (Jakobson and Halle 1956; Jakobson 1964). Applying this dichotomy to aphasia, he distinguishes two basic types depending on whether the major deficiency lies in combination (contiguity) and context or in selection (similarity) and substitution. These axes reflect the syntagmatic and paradigmatic relationships conceptualized by De Saussure (1916) and Hjelmslev (1953), a distinction which is particularly relevant to retraining of syntax. Therapists too often simply give object-naming tasks to agrammatic patients (a selection task) instead of concentrating on *combination* of available items. Beyn and Shokhor-Trotskaya (1966) maintain that this can actually cause an agrammatism. Selection and combination also operate at the segmental phonological level.

It is fundamental to the Structuralist approach that items owe their identity to meaning-differentiating features. Thus phonemes have value inasmuch as substitution of one phoneme for another in the same word-position affects meaning. This principle is fundamental to therapy. A phoneme such as /p/ is trained not only in terms of articulatory positioning or acoustic analysis, but also as a phonemic entity which semantically *contrasts* the word *pen* with *ten*, *hen*, etc., or *map* with *mat*. The same principle may be applied to syntactic or lexical units, which contrast with each other in the same 'slot' in the sentence/utterance—*is* contrasts with *was*, *cup* with *mug*, *jug* or *glass*. These are examples of paradigmatic substitutions. Therapy at the phonological level would include practice of distinctive features in minimal-pair words. Trim's (1965) *English Pronunciation Illustrated*, although not written with this type of learner in mind, contains not only amusing illustrations but rhymes for every English phoneme. The most comprehensive list of minimal pairs that the authors have found, however, is Rockey (1973).

Some remarks about therapy for word-retrieval and semantic reinforcement

Therapy for defects at the lexical level may take many forms. It is considered by some that the impairment is in retrieval and not in lexical storage. Constrained sentence-completion or cliché-completion is a technique widely practised by therapists to elicit immediate word-retrieval. The long-term effectiveness of this is, however, still doubtful. An evaluation of various forms of cue has been carried out by Rochford and Williams (1962, 1963, 1965) and others, including Hatfield, Howard, Barber, Jones and Morton (1977) and in this volume by Patterson, Purell and Morton (chapter 6). There is nothing especially linguistically-oriented about such techniques to facilitate word-finding, whose utility must ultimately rest on patients' abilities to provide the cue or strategy for themselves. Nevertheless, observation of some successful strategies, even if only temporary, as well as close study of paraphasias, paralexias and paragraphias, may throw light on the way in which the lexicon is organized.

A major contribution of Structural Linguistics has been the concept of a Semantic Field. The lexical stock can be seen to have its own system in which every item has its place in a network of other, semantically related, and perhaps phonologically related, lexical items. Items may be related in various ways— synonymy, antonymy, hierarchy (superordination), class membership. A type of Distinctive Feature analysis may be used, whereby lexical items are identified and contrasted by presence or absence of certain attributes, such as 'animate' versus 'inanimate' (this can be expressed as $+/-$ animate), 'edible' versus 'inedible', 'man-made' versus 'occurring in nature'. Sometimes one item of a contrasting pair may be perceived to be psychologically 'marked' and the other, generally the commoner one, 'unmarked'. Although somewhat outdated in theoretical linguistics, these concepts are used in neurolinguistics (Lesser 1978) and the authors believe them to be useful in therapy.

These relationships may sometimes be exploited in trying to help the patient to access certain items in his lexicon. Thus Seron, Deloche, Bastard, Chassin and Hermand (1979) found that when they drilled four patients in items from four semantic categories, i.e. clothes, house, tools and action verbs, all four improved in their retrieval of non-practised items in these categories and two showed significant improvement in finding lexical items in the two non-drilled categories of food and activities. This is similar to 'irradiation effects' (Weigl and Bierwisch, 1970). Marshall and Newcombe (1966) suggest that certain semantic confusions support the idea that a lexical entry is characterized by a set of semantic markers which indicate the general property of the word, plus a distinguisher indicating its idiosyncratic property. Brain damage thus results in an inability to retrieve these distinguishing features. Other researchers are now collecting evidence that in certain forms of aphasia semantic field organization becomes blurred and distorted (Goodglass and Baker 1976). Luria, Naydin, Tsvetkova and Vinarskaya (1969) have also commented on the limitation of word meanings and the conceptual structure of speech, and for certain groups of patient they actively attempt to reteach concepts.

Work on one aspect of language is often found to facilitate improvement at other levels, which highlights the importance of operating with larger units than the word, if possible. Semantic therapy includes identification and labelling of objects or concepts when the therapist draws attention to meaning-differentiating or meaning-integrating features. In planning therapy for syntax the semantics of words and sentence relations must be taken into account, as must pragmatic and functional aspects. It can be seen from the above that there is constant interaction between syntax and semantics. This is illustrated in some of the therapeutic techniques, which are described below.

An approach to the remediation of severe agrammatism

The severe agrammatism sometimes seen in Broca's aphasia can be tackled at the level of meaning relations or at the level of surface structure. The choice depends largely on the degree of impairment. Some cases strongly resist attempts of the therapist to improve the surface grammar. If a patient has lost so much of the surface structure that he or she is unable to convey verbally any structural notion of who is acting (the Agent) and what is being done (the Action), or if the patient's ability to organize his or her fragmentary utterances into some sort of Topic and Comment is impaired, then their greatest need is for a functional grammatical approach, sometimes referred to as semantically based grammar (Hatfield and Elvin 1978; Hatfield 1979). The patient must initially be helped to see that one-word utterances (even where the intent is to express a proposition) are often inadequate to convey a message. Practice is then given in expressing elementary propositions in response to thematic picture stimuli. The patient is required to produce structures which conform to some sort of primitive 'grammatical' system, even if it involves abnormal simplification and deletion. This presupposes possession of a small lexicon, initially composed of nouns, verbs or verbal forms (probably -ing forms), adjectives and adverbs. The immediate task is one of *combination* of appropriate lexical items. Structures such as 'gardener – digging', 'gardener – tired', 'table – old', 'table – broken', are accepted at this stage, especially when uttered with appropriate intonation. Verbal and adjectival forms are grouped together into one category. These combinations represent a direct advance on the mere labels 'gardener' and 'table', or even 'tired', where no proposition is expressed, unless the subject has been specified by the therapist ('What is the gardener feeling like?'). These two-word utterances are also preferred to combinations such as 'the gardener', or 'gardener is', or even 'is digging' on its own, although at some later stage such combinations might be practised to improve the melodic aspect. Omission of function words and occasionally of bound morphemes is not presented to the patient as an end in itself, or even as a model; what is stressed is the essential expression of the most meaningful conceptual items in the picture or situation and their relationship to each other. The principle here is that clause structure precedes phrase structure.

Introduction of prepositions and other function-word classes is delayed until there is sufficient facility with simple SV and SVO structures. Strategies such as replacement of locational prepositions by adverbs, verbs or nouns *functioning* as relational elements are also accepted at this stage, for example *cup up table*, or *cup top table* instead of *(the) cup (is) on (the) table*. Agrammatic patients often find such devices easier to produce than the normal form and there is no point in being purist while every 'complete' utterance is such an effort for the patient (Hatfield and Elvin 1978). Similar strategies include the use of free morphemes such as *now* or *soon* to replace conjugation of the verb as a tense marker. Such devices are constantly employed by some patients, more or less spontaneously, in addition to interrogative formulations such as 'Mrs Hatfield holiday, yes-no?', to replace the normal/acceptable interrogative transformation and (normal) use of the pronoun *you* in this context. Where the restoration of normal syntax is an unrealistic goal such strategies should be encouraged and reinforced and even on occasion introduced.

Therapy for patients with residual syntactic skills

Where more of the surface structure is regained fairly early and there are other good reasons for working directly on the surface structure, the customary procedure is followed of ascertaining which structures (and lexical items) are preserved and consolidating these and then building on them by expansion. For both approaches (working on surface structure or at a 'deeper' level) it is recognized that language is essentially dialogue and as soon as possible the emerging 'propositional' language, whether normal or simplified in its morphology, is incorporated into a discourse. Such practice in conversational situations, however limited the patient's verbal resources, will give experience in handling difficulties at the social and functional level, and heighten motivation and morale, since there is genuine communicative interaction.

For working on surface structure a small Manual has been developed proposing and illustrating a gradation of Basic Sentence Types. These begin with SVs, SVOs and SVCs (NP + cop + adj). After practising a few examples, patients are encouraged to look around them or at magazine pictures they themselves have chosen, and to add their own examples using their own lexicon, but modelled on target syntactic patterns. The Manual completes each Sentence-Type Unit with incorporation of the Sentence-Type into a dialogue showing how it might occur naturally in conversation (Hatfield 1979).

The essential difference between the two approaches rests on the assumption that in the first case grammatical function is severely to totally disrupted, in the second, that it is less severely impaired.

An extension of the idea of model sentence types and their occurrence in dialogue is carried over into a series of videotapes specially made in our department. The tapes portray scenes from everyday life as two or three characters engage in simple conversation—and occasionally argument—centred on their activities —making tea, going to the pub, watching television, visiting the supermarket, mending the bicycle, riding on a bus, and so on. At intervals the characters break off and address the audience/patients, prompting responses. Any semantically apposite response is welcomed, but the target or model responses are provided for guidance and are reinforced. The viewers/patients may be asked to recapitulate events or comments from the scene. Some of the questions are fairly open-ended. Others are much more convergent and in the early, most elementary scenes the questions are simply, 'what is this?', 'what is x doing?', 'what is x like?'. A major difference between this video series and the Manual is that the VTR programmes are less structured, although following a definite linguistic and psychological progression. They inherently represent both stimulation and revision of linguistic structures that are not lost but relatively unavailable, rather than retraining these. (There are also more structured VTR programmes, dealing with other 'levels' of language.)

The video-viewing is generally supervised by the therapist initially to ensure the patient's active participation but later on may be supervised by a volunteer helper or student. Many patients have been sufficiently motivated to work at the videotapes on their own, or with another patient. Role-play is another, and even more realistic, example of work at the level of functional communication. Most aphasic patients will take part in a non-threatening group round a table. One session, working on SVC and SVO structures caused great hilarity, when a Broca patient playing a consultant on a ward round produced utterances such as, 'she's very ill', 'man's got pneumonia', 'lady's had it!'.

Further material for structured work on syntax

The paucity of therapy material suitable for direct work on surface syntax, when drills or programmed structured exercises are indicated as part of the therapy plan, has led to the development of a more elaborate battery of materials. Using the system and terminology of '*The University Grammar of English*', (Quirk and Greenbaum 1973) a series of 'phrase structure envelopes' have been produced.

Each envelope contains 20 or so card realizations of a particular English phrase structure, ranging in length from one to several words. In the filing system, they are organized according to the number of words on the card, but this is not to suggest that this is a set order that must be followed with each patient. Each patient will have a different ability to select or sequence the cards, which are designed to be used in a variety of ways such as matching to pictures, reading aloud, sequencing into phrases or sentences, using them as answers to questions and so on.

While believing that no mass methods or materials are possible in aphasia therapy, the authors have nonetheless found it useful to be able to adapt a flexible general therapy material to an individual patient's therapy plan, using carefully selected items and techniques. This particular material is intended primarily for the Broca and non-fluent types of aphasic patient, but has also proved useful with other types.

Below is a brief summary, including examples, of the kind of 'immediate constituent' structures available.

One Word
Nouns	—	separate envelopes for singular and plural forms, and for animate and non-animate and proper nouns.
Lexical Verbs	—	all structural forms of many common verbs.
Adjectives	—	place, manner and time.
Auxiliaries	—	with, and without the contracted negative.
Pronouns	—	separate envelopes for each case paradigm.
Determiners		
Prepositions		
Question words		
Co-ordinators and subordinators		

Two-Word Examples
Determiner + Noun	—	again, a variety of noun type and form.
Adjective + Noun	—	"
Auxiliary + Verb	—	all structural forms of the verb that may occur with an auxiliary, both with and without negative particle.

Three-Word Examples
Determiner + Adjective + Noun.
Preposition + Adjective + Noun.

Four-Word Examples
Determiner + Intensifier + Adjective + Noun.
Preposition + Determiner + Adjective + Noun.

Miscellaneous Examples
Adverbial Clause	—	Finite and Non-Finite.
Relative Clause.		

Of course, the envelopes do not pretend to be a complete list of all types of simple English phrase structures, nor could they be. The material can be adapted to give greater specificity of—for example—verb-phrase syntactic structure, or semantic variation within the prepositional structures. Nouns can be subdivided according to characteristics such as frequency, or concreteness, or to take into account their phonological structure.

Thus a wide variety of lexical items can be selected by the therapist to act as clause-structure realizations in the Subject, Verb, Object, Complement or Adverbial 'slots' of practice sentences. For example, a Subject might be realized by any one of these structures. (Several examples of each multi-word structure to illustrate the different noun types used.)

Noun (Proper)	e.g.	Mrs Thatcher
Noun (human-plural)	e.g.	lawyers
Noun (animal-plural)	e.g.	cows
Noun (inanimate-plural)	e.g.	bricks
Pronoun (subjective case)	e.g.	he
Adjective + Noun	e.g.	outspoken Benn, tired doctors, sick sheep, fine buildings.
Determiner + Noun	e.g.	the President, my representative, those horses, her lectures.
Determiner + Adjective + Noun	e.g.	the original City, her strong sons, some poor giraffes, no evening meals.
Adjective + Adjective + Noun	e.g.	dirty old Soho, tall handsome actors, cold hungry herds, long boring stories.

These few examples show a little of the variety of structures and realizations which are possible for any sequencing work using this material. Whenever possible patients are encouraged to participate as partners in their therapy plans, and personalized realizations are always added to the drill material. For a keen cricketer, the Determiner + Adjective + Noun envelope also contained items such as, 'the famous Boycott', 'the English team', 'that cunning bowler' and 'their best batsman'.

Although not all patients can read the cards initially, much therapy work utilizes written language to help spoken, and the therapist would encourage recognition of word cards before any sequencing work was begun. The 'structure envelopes' can act as a model on which to base any structured spoken work, even if reading is not possible. Work is in progress with the help of other therapists to produce pictures specifically for work on clause and phrase structures.

Using the general principles outlined earlier in this chapter, and having carefully assessed the patient's phonological, lexical and syntactic ability, appropriate structures and therapy tasks would be selected. Just one concrete example follows: with a non-fluent patient, who is producing single-word utterances only, it might seem appropriate to work on expansion of utterances from one to two elements. A plan might include work on the following:

(Subject + Verb) = Proper Noun + Verb, 3rd person singular;
(Subject + Verb) = Noun (plural) + Verb, base form;
(Verb + Object) = Verb (Base) + Noun (plural);
(Verb + Adverbial) = Verb (Base) + Adverb (manner);
(Verb + Complement) = Verb ('be' form) + Adjective;
(Adjective + Noun).

The wide variety of lexical items in each envelope ensures that a range of grammatical sentences can be generated, with the patient needing to choose appropriate, meaningful combinations.

This can also be useful for the fluent, Wernicke-type patient. Mrs N.D. (described above) needed much work to help her to recognize and control her speech flow. Using highly constrained sentence frames, she practised constructing semantically meaningful sequences of items, reading them aloud and judging their semantic acceptability before writing them down herself. For example, a variety of sentences can be generated by selecting only three realizations of each of these structures:

Determiner + Adjective + Noun (human) e.g. the old politician,
   the famous boxer,
   my older brother.

Determiner + Adjective + Noun (inanimate) e.g. a cold potato,
   the heavy door,
   his grimy hands.

Verb (past)   e.g. ate,
   flattened,
   washed.

Only a few are meaningful.

Flexible and imaginative use of the syntax material does not result in patient boredom, but allows programmed work to be easily produced. The authors have found that patients, their relatives and volunteers all enjoy this kind of work, and understand clearly the rationale behind it.

Concluding remarks

It is only by describing aims and methods precisely that the efficacy of speech therapy for aphasia can truly be evaluated. Too many papers gloss over the details of the therapeutic programme, so that objective judgement of its actual relevance to improvement in the patient's language function is virtually impossible. The usefulness of different methods and assumptions of therapy must be tested, since, as Hegde, Noll and Pecora (1979) note, 'in the final analysis, the generalization of trained verbal responses applied to novel, untrained situations, persons and linguistic contexts is what determines the effectiveness of a language programme' (p. 301). Linguistics fosters the specification and planning of appropriate and effective language remediation. Nevertheless, the full extent of its efficacy and its utility to other therapists depends on provision of a detailed account of every therapeutic step undertaken and rigorous pre- and post-testing.

However great the need to apply linguistic science to the analysis of aphasic speech and to the planning of any remediation, it is important not to regard the use of linguistics as a panacea for treatment. Indeed, it could be misleading to rely on the findings of linguistics alone, without concurrently examining for a multitude of possible disturbances—of perception, attention, orientation, cognition or memory. Moreover, although the discipline of linguistics can identify aspects and degree of language breakdown and give guidelines as to the direction that therapy should take and the order in which items and structures should be practised, it cannot specify learning strategies. Linguistics, in collaboration with psycholinguistics and cognitive psychology, can contribute a great deal to the understanding of *what* to train and *how* learning or re-learning can best be achieved.

This chapter has suggested some ways in which linguistics might be directly applied to the analysis and planning of appropriate therapy in aphasia. The next decade will certainly see further systematic applications of different aspects of this discipline by aphasia therapists. Particularly to be anticipated are developments in the investigation of prosodic factors in comprehension and production and in the application of discourse analysis. Such developments will help to fill some of the many gaps in planning therapy for aphasic patients.

Acknowledgements
We wish to express our gratitude to the Consultants of Addenbrooke's Hospital who have encouraged the research and development aspects of our Department and given us much practical and personal support; also to our patients, some of whom have acted willingly and good-humouredly as 'guinea-pigs' while we have been developing new techniques and materials; and finally to our colleagues in linguistics and psychology, Dr M. Garman and Dr J. Morton for their much needed criticism of our ideas.

6
Facilitation of word retrieval in aphasia
Karalyn Patterson, Christina Purell and John Morton

Introduction

The late John C. Ogilvie, Professor of Psychology and Statistics at the University of Toronto, had a sign in his office which read: 'If you torture the data long enough, they will confess anything'. Some people might use much the same description to characterize the intentions and/or techniques of experimental psychologists who work with aphasic patients: 'If you torture the patients long enough, they will provide data to support your theory'. Of course, this is in jest: the patients who provided the present data were tested therapeutically, and they enjoyed participating in the study. More apposite here, however, is the fact that the results obtained disprove the maxim: the patients, though tested long enough, did not confess the answers that were sought.

The main question asked, motivated both by its therapeutic and its theoretical implications, was this: If an aphasic patient has difficulty (as almost all patients do, with some degree of severity) in finding a word or name for something, can one demonstrate the effectiveness of techniques intended to ameliorate this difficulty? In particular we were concerned with relatively long-term benefits to word retrieval. From the available literature as well as from observations of our own and of our speech therapist colleagues, it was expected that various techniques would facilitate immediate word retrieval. Pease Myers and Goodglass (1978), for example, evaluated phonemic cueing (or 'first sounds', as they label this technique, e.g. providing the patient with the spoken cue 'la' when he is trying to name a picture of a ladder); all diagnostic categories of aphasic patients showed significant facilitation in naming given this type of cue. Having received the cue and successfully named the object, however, will the patient show an increased probability of correctly naming a ladder if asked to do so ten minutes or half an hour later? This question, the answer to which is much less apparent from the literature, was the focus of this research.

There are, as always, at least some published data germane to the present study. The discussion of these data will be delayed until later in the chapter, when the present methods and results will have been described and can more easily be compared with previous findings.

Two studies will be reported here, one each to evaluate repetition and phonemic cueing as techniques with potential long-term beneficial effects on word retrieval. Picture naming constituted the experimental task in both studies. Although naming may be a limited aspect of language, it is also a prominent one whose disruption is (as every therapist knows) enormously frustrating to patients. The therapeutic implications of the research thus need no justification or even explication. Theoretically, naming performance by aphasic patients can provide important input to our understanding of certain cognitive and linguistic processes both in their normal and their impaired modes of operation.

Subjects

Since patients of the same type (and in some cases the same patients) participated in Experiments 1 and 2, this section refers to both studies. The subjects were all adult neurological patients (typically with vascular aetiology) obtained through the services of one of the speech-therapy departments in East Anglia, the majority through Addenbrooke's Hospital, Cambridge. The primary criterion for inclusion in the sample was that the patient should demonstrate a significant naming or word-finding deficit, defined as at least 15 per cent failures on a screening test of picture naming. Additional criteria, some rather intuitively assessed, included the facts that the patient should (a) be at least three months post CVA; (b) have no severe visual problems; (c) be able to understand and follow the experimental instructions; (d) have no notable difficulty in repetition of single words; and (e) have no difficulty in recognizing and understanding drawings of common objects. By this final criterion, it was intended to restrict the phenomenon being studied to deficits of naming or word retrieval rather than agnosic difficulties. On any particular occasion that a patient fails to name an object, it may of course be difficult to know whether the failure is one of recognition or naming. There are however empirical means to enable basic discrimination between these problems (see Caramazza and Berndt 1978, and Saffran 1982, for discussions of this question); and in practice the nature of the patient's error response often provides the basis for an informed judgement (Lesser 1978, 75–6).

Application of the above criteria, plus the requirement that the patients be regularly available for the weeks needed for assessment and full testing, yielded a total sample of 14 patients for Experiment 1 and 11 for Experiment 2. By the Boston Diagnostic Aphasia Examination (Goodglass and Kaplan 1972), the patient sample could be roughly characterized as about one-half anomic aphasics and one-quarter each Broca's and Wernicke's aphasics.

Materials

The stimulus materials for both experiments consisted of a set of 265 unambiguous pen and ink drawings of objects, each on a $3\frac{1}{2}$" $\times$ $5\frac{1}{2}$" white card. The pictures were selected from a much larger set on the basis that, in a pre-test, at least 90 per cent of a group of 40 normal subjects provided the same name for each of these 265 drawings.

The names of the objects covered a wide range of frequency of occurrence in written English (Kučera and Francis 1967). Wherever subsets of words were subjected to different experimental treatment, care was taken to balance the subsets for frequency since it is well known that this variable can influence success in object naming (e.g. Rochford and Williams 1965; Wiegel-Crump and Koenigsknecht 1973).

Experiment 1: repetition

The general issue of interest, whether difficult words become easier to retrieve as a result of repetition, was translated into several experimental questions. Firstly, the expectation was that repetition of a word would facilitate an immediately subsequent attempt to retrieve that name in response to a picture. Secondly, it is logical that this beneficial influence should decrease with time and/or other events intervening between repetition and naming; but how rapidly does it decrease and, most importantly, does measurable facilitation remain after some 'sensible' period of time? For example, would it be possible (in a speech therapy session) to return to a difficult word which had been repeated 15 or 30 minutes earlier, and expect to find some residual effect upon which to build? Thirdly, do multiple repetitions produce a stronger or more lasting effect than a single repetition? And finally, if multiple repetitions are given, are they differentially effective as a function of their spacing, e.g. five repetitions of a particular word in immediate succession compared with five repetitions spread out by intervening events?

Design

For each patient, certain words were selected as target (difficult) words on the basis of naming performance on a pre-test with the 265 pictures. Five target words were assigned to condition R + N (Repetition plus Naming) and five to condition N (Naming alone); for six consecutive trials of an identical pattern, naming performance was compared for these two conditions. The pattern of a trial is displayed in Table 6.1 using a sample set of picture names. In the first phase of the trial, the patient engaged in one repetition each of 26 words, only five of which (those labelled R + N) are pertinent for the moment. In the second phase of the trial, the patient was tested on naming 26 pictures. The last five picture names, targets $N_1 - N_5$, had received no repetition in the first phase, and the patient's performance on these targets is to be compared with performance on the R + N target words which *were* repeated in phase 1. Furthermore, note from Table 1 that the R + N words in the naming phase were tested in the reverse order to their occurrence in the repetition phase. Since the naming test followed the repetition phase immediately, this means that nothing intervened between repetition of word $R + N_5$ and the naming test on picture $R + N_5$; ten events (five repetitions and five naming attempts on other words) intervened between repetition and naming of $R + N_4$; 40 events intervened between repetition and naming of $R + N_1$. The words in Table 1 printed in lower case were filler items serving two purposes. Firstly, they allowed us to space the R + N target items to achieve lags of 0, 10, 20, 30 and 40 items intervening between repetition and naming. Secondly, these filler items were

FACILITATION OF WORD RETRIEVAL IN APHASIA

Table 6.1 A sample of the basic pattern for trials 1–6 in Experiment 1

REPETITION		NAMING TEST		
$R-SP_1$	ROCKET	$R+N_5$	GATEPOST	(lag 0)
$R-SP_2$	MAYOR		boy	
$R-SP_3$	SUITCASE		goat	
$R-SP_4$	COW		eggs	
$R-SP_5$	BLOUSE		Indian	
$R+N_1$	BOW	$R+N_4$	TOE	(lag 10)
	boy		teeth	
	goat		king	
	eggs		watch	
	Indian		duck	
$R+N_2$	TABLE	$R+N_3$	STETHOSCOPE	(lag 20)
	teeth		butter	
	king		thermometer	
	watch		crab	
	duck		shoe	
$R+N_3$	STETHOSCOPE	$R+N_2$	TABLE	(lag 30)
	butter		dice	
	thermometer		igloo	
	crab		face	
	shoe		tea	
$R+N_4$	TOE	$R+N_1$	BOW	(lag 40)
	dice	N_1	SKIRT	
	igloo	N_2	PROPELLOR	
	face	N_3	TANK	
	tea	N_4	PATH	
$R+N_5$	GATEPOST	N_5	GLOBE	

names which the patient had successfully retrieved on the pre-test; since they were probably somewhat easier for the patient than the target items, their inclusion should ensure that the naming test on each trial consisted of many successes as well as some failures.

The remaining upper-case words in Table 1, labelled R-SP (Repetition—Spaced), represent one of three other types of target word conditions. The five R-SP words were repeated once each at the beginning of trials 1–5, but no naming test was given for these words until trial 6. R-SP target words thus received five repetitions, spaced out over the test session, prior to the presentation of the appropriate pictures for naming. For the two remaining target conditions, all repetition and naming components occurred entirely within trial 6. At the *beginning* of trial 6, prior to the normal pattern of events displayed in Table 1, five target words in condition MR-DEL (Massed Repetition—Delayed) were repeated. Each word was repeated five times in immediate succession (hence, Massed); the naming test on these words came at the end of trial 6 (hence, Delayed). *After* the basic unit of events on trial 6, five target words in condition MR-IMM (Massed Repetition

—Immediate) were first repeated five times each and then tested immediately by asking for the relevant pictures to be named.

Trials 1–6 constituted a single test session, involving 25 target words (five each in five target conditions) and 16 filler words. Each patient participated in a total of three such test sessions, with a new set of target and filler words for each session.

Procedure

In the pre-test session, each patient attempted to name the 265 stimulus pictures. Pictures correctly named within 5 sec. were assigned to the pool of items from which that patient's filler words would be drawn; pictures not correctly named within 5 sec. became target items. A period of approximately one week elapsed before the first experimental session and also before each subsequent session. Each of the three experimental sessions consisted of six trials, each trial with repetition and naming phases as described previously. During repetition phases, the patient was simply asked to repeat the appropriate words after the speech threapist; during the naming phases, the patient was given 5 sec., without any assistance, to name each picture. All responses were written down by the therapist and tape recorded as well in case of ambiguity.

Results

Consider first the general contrast between performance on N words (which the patient simply attempted to name for six trials) and on R + N words (which the patient repeated and then attempted to name for six trials). The two main data functions for trials 1–6 in Figure 6.1 present the relevant observations, combined over the three sessions per patient and (for the moment) over the varying lags between repetition and naming in condition R + N. The short-term beneficial effect of repetition is immediately apparent: probability of correct naming was consistently higher in condition R + N than in condition N. However it is also clear that this effect showed no increment with successive trials: although the same words were repeated and named six times, the advantage of R + N over N was no greater on trial 6 than on trial 1.

Figure 6.1 also shows the results on trial 6 for the three other target conditions, where five repetitions of the target words occurred before the appropriate naming tests. These conditions assessed both the spacing of the repetitions and the delay between repetitions and test; the results suggest that only the latter factor is critical. Five massed repetitions substantially facilitated naming performance when the naming test occurred immediately after the repetitions. Given any appreciable delay between repetition and naming, however, (a) the massed-spaced variable had no significant effect; and (b) for both conditions, performance was no better (in fact slightly worse) than naming after a single repetition (e.g. R + N on trial 1).

Returning to the R + N results, the data function in Figure 6.1 is a composite of different lags between repetition and naming on each trial. The analysis as a function of lag appears in Figure 6.2, combined over trials 1–6 since (as is obvious from

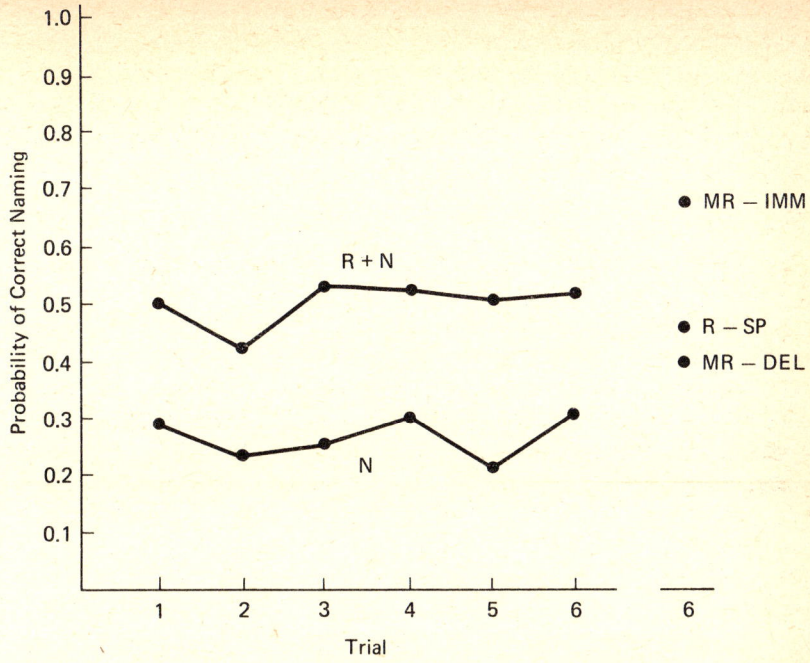

Figure 6.1 The mean probability of a patient correctly naming a drawing in the various conditions. N—Control naming condition; R + N—prior repetition of the name; MR–IMM—massed name repetition with immediate naming trial; MR–DEL—massed name repetition with delayed naming trial; R–SP—spaced repetition practice with subsequent naming trial.

Figure 6.1) no significant changes occurred over trials. Figure 6.2 demonstrates what one might have guessed from the absence of cumulative effects in Figure 6.1: the benefit from repetition was a decreasing function of delay. When no events intervened between repetition and naming, performance was greatly enhanced (about .70 correct naming as contrasted with about .30 in condition N). Measurable benefit was still present after 10 or 20 intervening events; but by the time that 30 intervening events had elapsed, the probability of correct naming (about .40) was only slightly higher than naming in the absence of repetition. Given the design of the experiment, the results are properly analysed in terms of number of intervening events rather than time. To give a rough impression of the time scale, however (and with the caveat that time varied from patient to patient, from trial to trial, and even within a trial), lag 30 perhaps represents a delay of about four or five minutes.

The results across various target conditions were surprisingly consistent, and can be summarized as follows. For this group of patients and this set of target words, naming in the absence of any facilitating technique has a probability of success of around .30 (condition N). Given one or more repetitions *immediately* before naming, this probability rises to around .70 (condition R + N lag 0 and condition

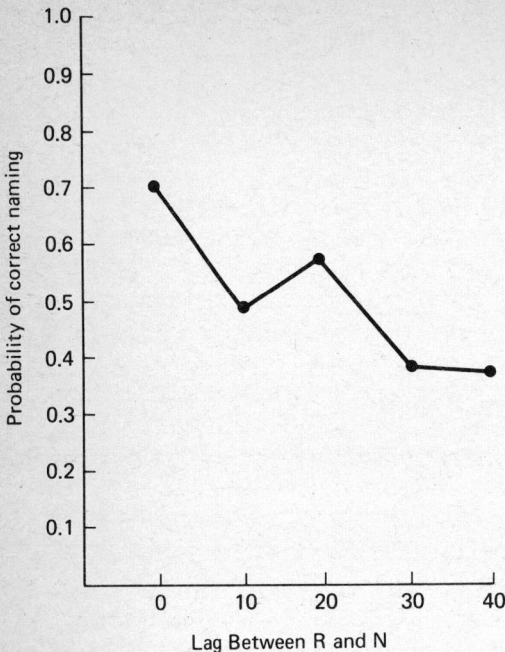

Figure 6.2 The effects of the lag between the repetition trial and the naming trial on naming performance.

MR-IMM). Given any appreciable delay between the repetition(s) and naming, the probability of success returns to around .40 (condition R + N lags 30 and 40, condition MR-DEL and condition R-SP). While these values are not quite back to the baseline value of .30, neither do they represent a notable advantage. Furthermore, the absence of cumulative effects or 'learning' is particularly disappointing. For specific R + N words, this can be shown by the conditional probability that a particular word will be named correctly on a particular trial given that it was failed on the preceding trial. On trial 2 (the first one, obviously, where such an analysis is possible), the probability of correct naming for words failed on trial 1 was .07 for condition N and .24 for condition R + N. (Performance for R + N was of course higher than N because the R + N words had just been repeated). If repetition produced some lasting and cumulative effect, then over trials one would expect this conditional probability to rise for condition R + N while remaining unchanged for condition N. The probability of correct naming on trial 5 for words failed on trial 4, however, was .08 for condition N and .27 for condition R + N. Although the R + N words had by this point been repeated five times, they were no more likely to move from failed to successful status than at the beginning of the session.

Experiment 2: phonemic cueing

As for repetition in the first study, the expectation was that a phonemic cue for a difficult-to-retrieve word would facilitate the patient's immediate attempt at naming. The primary question was whether word retrieval would still show measurable benefit some time after the phonemic cueing procedure. In addition the effects of two different forms of phonemic cueing were also assessed.

Design

Unlike Experiment 1 where target words were identified in a separate pre-test session, Experiment 2 involved a sort of on-line procedure whereby failed words in the naming test were immediately (that is, after 5 sec.) assigned to one of three conditions. In the Control condition, to provide a baseline for the additional time and effort that would be devoted to words in the two experimental cueing conditions, patients were simply encouraged to go on trying to retrieve the name for the picture, for a total of 20 sec., without any direct assistance from the therapist. In the Repeated Cue condition, the therapist produced the initial sound or phoneme of the word (e.g. /tə/ for 'telephone') and repeated this single cue up to three times, once every 5 sec., if the patient continued to be unable to retrieve the object name. In the Progressive Cue condition, the initial cue gave the first sound only, exactly as in the Repeated condition; but each subsequent cue added additional phonemic information (e.g. for 'telephone': (1) /tə/, (2) /te/, (3) /tel/). Approximately one-third of the words that each patient failed to name were assigned to each of the three conditions in rotation. Thirty minutes after the end of the cueing phase, the entire set of pictures was re-presented for naming to allow comparison between previously cued and non-cued words.

Procedure

Each patient was in fact tested on the set of picture names three times in the experiment, twice on the day of the cueing procedure (as described above) and once three weeks earlier for a general assessment of performance. On the first and third of these tests, the patient was simply presented with each picture for 5 sec.; if the patient named it, the speech therapist proceeded to the next picture; if the patient failed to name it, the therapist said the name and then went on to the next picture. On the second test, which incorporated the cueing procedure, the patient was instructed that assistance would be given on some of the difficult words. For failed words assigned to the Control condition, the patient was merely encouraged to continue efforts to retrieve the picture name. For failed words assigned to one of the cueing conditions, the appropriate cues were presented. If the patient produced the correct name at any point, the therapist went on to the next item; otherwise the cueing proceeded to the third and final one. There then followed a 30-minute interval which was filled with general chat and a cup of coffee, following which the entire set of pictures were re-presented for naming. In all cases, the speech therapist both wrote and tape-recorded all responses.

Results

The total proportions of pictures correctly named within 5 sec. and without assistance on the three occasions were as follows: three weeks before the cueing procedure, .42; during the cueing procedure (that is, before any cues were offered), .43; half an hour after the cueing procedure, .45. These values are indicative both of the severity and the stability of the patients' naming deficits. These overall values also provide a hint that the cueing procedure had no long-term effect; however this question must be evaluated in terms of specific words subjected to specific treatments.

For an assessment, first, of the immediate effectiveness of phonemic cueing, the centre section of Table 6.2 shows performance on Control and Cued words. All of these words of course failed to be produced in the first 5 sec. of the picture's presentation. In a total of 20 sec., without assistance, .20 of the Control words were successfully retrieved. Thus further time and effort by the patient did yield success on a small proportion of items. By contrast, the cueing procedure was dramatically effective: given a single cue and only 5 sec. additional time (thus, after 10 sec.), naming performance had achieved twice the rate of the Control words after 20 sec.; given two or three cues at successive 5-sec. intervals, the advantage of Cued words over the Control words was even more impressive.

Table 6.2 also reveals the large expected difference between Repeated and Progressive cueing. The patients clearly could make effective use of the additional phonemic information provided in the Progressive condition; by the time that a cue containing three phonemes of the target word had been offered, the patients were able to produce the majority of names. It is interesting to note that, in the Repeated condition, a second repetition of the same single-phoneme cue produced at least a small advantage over just one presentation, though there was little further increment between two and three repetitions of the same cue. For a person with unimpaired naming skills, 5 sec. would be a very long period of time either as a naming latency or as a time required for some manipulation to produce its effect. For aphasic patients, however, even when a procedure like cueing does benefit word retrieval, it seems that the patient may require an abnormal length of time to take advantage of the cue.

Table 6.2 Probability of correct naming in the various conditions of Experiment 2

	3 weeks earlier	\multicolumn{4}{c}{*During Cueing*}	*30 min. later*
		5	10	within 15	20 sec	
Control	.11	.00			.20	.25
Cued	.28	.00	.40	.53 / .70	.58 Rep / .87 Prog	.25
			(1st)	(2nd)	(3rd) Cue	

The next question is whether the impressive short-term facilitation from phonemic cueing survives any delay between cueing and naming. Table 6.2 provides two contrasts germane to this issue. Firstly, if the cueing procedure produced some durable trace, then 30 minutes later, naming performance on the *Cued* words should have been superior to that on *Control* words. Performance on these specific subsets of words in the delayed test, shown at the right-hand side of Table 6.2, reveals no hint of such an effect. Secondly, if cueing produced any lasting effect, then performance on the *Cued* words 30 minutes after cueing should have been superior to performance on the *same* subset of words within the whole set tested three weeks earlier. Table 6.2 reveals that for these words, performance on the delayed test after cueing (.25) showed no hint of benefit relative to the test several weeks before cueing (.28). Thus, while confirming that phonemic cueing is effective at the time of its administration, no evidence has been obtained for its longer-term efficacy.

General discussion

The results must now be interpreted in terms of other relevant research on this issue, as well as therapeutic and theoretical implications. As noted in our introduction, there is not a great deal in the existing literature on aphasia to indicate whether one ought to expect the kind of lasting facilitation which was sought but failed to emerge. There are however at least three studies showing improvements in naming performance under somewhat different conditions, from which positive results in the current study might have been predicted.

Hatfield, Howard, Barber, Jones and Morton (1977) studied naming by aphasic patients of real objects and line drawings. Hatfield *et al*. obtained an effect of repeated occurrence of the same object for naming. On three successive tests on a small set of objects, the proportion of correct naming rose from .51 to .60 to .67. This rise in performance with successive tests or trials is what conspicuously failed to emerge in Experiment 1. Several differences between the two studies may account for the apparent discrepancy in results. Most importantly, in the previous study the average lag between two successive tests on a given object was 6 intervening items. With lags of 0 or 10 items between repetition and naming, the present study also found facilitation of naming. It is therefore predicted that in a procedure virtually identical to that used by Hatfield *et al*. but with increased spacing between successive tests, their incremental effect would disappear.

Weigl (1961, 1970) described the phenomenon of deblocking of responses in an impaired modality by use of a different modality which is either intact or at least less severely impaired. Translated into the present context, this might mean that the patient's ability to repeat a word (Experiment 1) or use a phonemic cue to retrieve a word (Experiment 2) should have facilitated any subsequent attempt to produce that word in response to a picture. Two crucial factors may explain why this is not in fact a justified prediction from Weigl's results to the present one. Firstly, there is once again the issue of the time course of such effects: note that Weigl (1961) called it 'the phenomenon of temporary deblocking'. Both of our techniques were notably successful on a temporary basis. Secondly, as Lesser (1978, 87) points out, Weigl's interpretation of deblocking (1970) is in terms of semantics or comprehension. The response failure is thought to derive from a comprehension problem which can then be overcome because a different modality does enable comprehension of the relevant word. In the present study, the impression was gained that the patients' failures in picture naming were not primarily attributable to comprehension deficits (partly of course because any patient for whom this did appear to be a major feature was excluded from the sample). There is a controversy (which cannot be entered into here) regarding the existence of *pure* anomia, with perfectly normal intact comprehension (see Lesser 1978, chapter 5 for discussion). It is not possible to insist that the patients used in the present study should be thus characterized; it is only possible to claim that, relatively speaking, their problem was more one of achieving access to the object's name than of access to the semantics of the object. Thus the phenomenon of deblocking may not be especially relevant here.

Wiegel-Crump and Koenigsknecht (1973) gave extensive practice (18 therapy sessions) on subsets of words which four aphasic patients had failed to name in a pre-test. After each block of six therapy sessions, picture naming was measured both on the practised items and on previously failed items which had received no training. All four patients showed dramatic improvements in naming of both trained and untrained items; from the data presented by Wiegel-Crump and Koenigsknecht (Table II, p. 416) it appears that the gains in proportion correct were greater on practised than on unpractised items, but the authors do not in fact report that this was a significant difference. Their therapy techniques were varied and multi-dimensional and included both of the procedures studied here (repetition and phonemic cueing) plus additional methods (e.g. supplying gestures, associated words and synonyms). Of the possible reasons for the discrepancy between this study and the present one, the richness and complexity of their therapeutic programme is the most likely. As with the Weigl studies, the involvement of 'central' factors contrasts starkly with the purely phonological techniques which have been evaluated here.

The finding of Wiegel-Crump and Koenigsknecht of substantial improvement on *untrained* items addresses an important theoretical issue. To what extent are the various deficits observed in aphasia specific to certain *items*, or characteristics of *processes* (and thus observable on any words or items)? The results of the Wiegel-Crump and Koenigsknecht study, if replicable, imply that at least for certain combinations of deficit and remedial programme, it is possible to facilitate not just the retrieval of specific items but the retrieval process itself. Such a conclusion would narrow the possible interpretations of the functional locus for anomia. A naming impairment which results from a deficit at the level of particular semantic representations should be restricted to individual items or groups of items (Warrington 1975). Improvements in the *general* retrievability of items then would argue against a semantic locus for the deficit. A naming impairment resulting from either (a) a prevailing impediment to the transmission of information from the semantic system to the output system, or (b) universally augmented thresholds on output devices, would give rise to non-specific effects, spanning all items (Morton and Patterson 1980a). It is far from clear by what mechanism(s) therapy would, respectively, (a) facilitate the transmission process or (b) reduce thresholds for the whole output system. But supposing such mechanisms do exist, the general improvement claimed by Wiegel-Crump and Koenigsknecht would be consistent with deficits of these sorts.

In the present study, of course, no persisting improvement was found even for practised items; our results thus require a different theoretical interpretation, to account for exclusively temporary changes in retrievability. There seem to be two options available. The first is that the short-term facilitation observed is due to changes in the availability of phonological output devices—termed the output logogen system in Morton and Patterson (1980a). For a variety of reasons, such facilitation would be expected to be relatively short-lived, unlike the results found with the equivalent input devices. The latter show modality-specific facilitation effects at least 45 minutes after a first presentation of an item—word or picture (Murrell and Morton 1974; Warren and Morton 1982). The current findings, then, could be seen as indicating directly the duration of output-facilitation effects. The alternative account is that the data should be seen as reflecting short-term episodic memory for a particular phonological code. This form of memory is probably not especially tenable beyond a minute or so, nor would it be easily convertible into a more lasting representation.

In concluding, the disappointing but unambiguous nature of the present findings must be emphasized. There is no doubt about the efficacy of the techniques evaluated here if one means *immediate* efficacy. To give a very rough summary of the results across all conditions of both experiments: for a set of difficult-to-retrieve names, the probability of our patients correctly producing such names was about .25 in the absence of assistance, but about .55 after a minimal phonemic cue, about .85 after an extensive phonemic cue and about .70 after one or more repetitions of the word. At the time of word-finding difficulty, these cueing techniques are highly effective. The testimony sought from our patients was evidence that some of this facilitation might survive beyond the immediate situation, but this they would not confess.

One final note: by no means can it be concluded that these techniques, successful in the short term, are without utility or should be abandoned. Dimensions which are considerably more difficult to measure than simple probability correct, such as the patient's self-confidence or release from frustration, may well benefit significantly from these procedures. As yet, however, no evidence has been obtained for their specific effectiveness in facilitating word retrieval.

Acknowledgements
This research was supported by a project grant from the Department of Health and Social Security. We are grateful to (1) the Department of Neurological Surgery and Neurology, Addenbrooke's Hospital, Cambridge, who provided facilities for and encouragement of our work; (2) the many Speech Therapy Departments in East Anglia who provided access to our patients; and (3) our patients.

Psychosocial Perspectives

The chapters in this section examine psychosocial and naturalistic aspects of aphasia therapy and what emerges is the growing relevance of this perspective to management. Brumfitt and Clarke describe a psychotherapeutic approach to psychosocial adjustment which emphasizes the need that the aphasic individual has for support and guidance through a traumatic experience. Müller and Code examine the perceptions of psychosocial adjustment to aphasia by the patient, significant individuals in the patient's life as well as by the therapist. More naturalistic and less clinically based approaches to therapy are discussed by Fawcus and by Meikle and Wechsler. Fawcus puts the case for a more socially based group-treatment approach and Meikle and Wechsler discuss the use of non-professional volunteers in more naturalistic settings.

7

An application of psychotherapeutic techniques to the management of aphasia

Shelagh Brumfitt and Peter Clarke

The two components of therapy

When working with dysphasic patients, speech therapists may often experience an uncomfortable conflict between their professional roles and their personal feelings. Their professional role is clearly to treat the presenting language disorder, which is what they are trained and employed to do. However, they are also sensitive to the distress, the confusion and isolation these people experience and may also want to respond to these needs. The difficulty is that these two roles often seem to compete for clinical time.

One way to resolve the conflict is to recognize that *most* treatments have two such components and that you cannot do one without the other. There is nearly always a technical component: for example linguistic exercises are used by speech therapists, drugs by physicians. There is *always* a personal interactional component. Whatever the profession, one person is potentially offering (or witholding, or making conditions about) some sort of good the other person is thought to need. You are 'doing something about it' both when you are giving technical help *and* when you are offering comfort, structure and understanding. Quite often, giving the personal help is a necessary first step before the patient is able to accept the technical help.

Speech therapy then, can in certain instances be seen as a special case of the general art of psychotherapy since it shares some common methods and aims with psychotherapy. It uses selected psychological methods; it pays attention to both verbal and nonverbal communications; and it aims to improve the free flow of communication between the patient and others by modelling and developing these skills of communication together in the treatment room.

As soon as any treatment begins, many memories will be triggered in both parties. There may well be both happy and disastrous memories of things that went right and went wrong when other people gave, received, cared for and accepted care. These memories will be woven together into the therapeutic relationship of the present. The expectations arising from these memories may here be disconfirmed, sometimes joyfully, sometimes sadly: sometimes they may be yet again tragically validated. The case is even clearer when the therapist works with a newly dysphasic patient. Here one person is faced with a major readjustment in life following a very traumatic and unforeseen experience, and the other person offers a substantial amount of time regularly in privacy and intimacy trying to be helpful over a period of months or even years. A good deal of treatment explicitly labelled psychotherapy is less intimate and extensive than this.

The development of individual identity

Before making suggestions about how to make the most of this psychotherapeutic challenge, it may be helpful to discuss ways of looking at man in general and people with dysphasia in particular. A valuable approach can be found in Kelly's Personal Construct Theory (Kelly 1955; Bannister and Mair 1968; Bannister and Fransella 1980). Kelly saw the person as a constantly changing (growing, decaying) set of processes, not as a static machine which has to be powered or kicked into activity and change, but as a natural flow. 'The person is not an object which is temporarily in a moving state but is himself a form of motion' (Kelly 1955, 48). Since this is a rather breathless, hectic way to live, Kelly thought that we try to deal with it by adopting the posture of natural scientists who try to understand the world by studying how to predict, or rather, anticipate events. We make these predictions about what is going to happen next by trying to see what happened in similar circumstances before, and making the bet that it will happen again. In order not to keep on losing our bets, we each of us work out more or less sophisticated form books (or scientific texts or technological manuals) based on all the transactions that have impinged on us in the past.

The major part of such a form book or manual is concerned with what happens in those interactions in which we personally participate, so it is devoted to the understanding and the prediction of our own behaviour, that is, what makes me *me*, an individual with my own identity. Although it is convenient to have 'a skin for keeping us in' a person is not bounded by his or her skin but is a social creation, a being defined by the set of role relationships in which he or she takes part. A simple illustration of this point is the way people readily offer a list of such role titles if you keep on asking them who they are: I am the spouse of, child of, parent of, teacher of, or I am a speech therapist, a psychologist, your boss, etc. It is reasonable to assume then that most of us maintain a sizeable proportion of ourselves in such relationships, of which we see ourselves as only parts rather than wholes.

It is considered that this view of ourselves as essentially social beings, belonging to, forming part of others, develops from our earliest experiences, and our sense of personal identity/individuality grows from a process of gradual discrimination. Parent-child interaction is now clearly established as starting in the first weeks of life and it may be that we find out 'who we are' (that is, become conscious of being a separate self) by gradually noticing the limits of our own effectiveness, where our feelings and intentions and physical movements stop changing and affecting things. At first there is perhaps very little sense of a difference between inside and outside of the skin, perhaps there is only what an adult would describe as *us*. Gradually as he or she grows, the baby's understanding and acquaintance widen, and the discovery is made that there is not one *us* but many *us's*. The *me* probably gradually emerges as the one common element in all these *us's*, the only bit that never goes away, the residue. The *others* are the bits that go to and fro, sometimes here, often not. In this way perhaps the *us's* split up into individual people. Of course this takes a lot of time and continues to develop long after the infant can use words like *me*, *you*, and *us* correctly.

To some extent the process goes on right through life: gradually as our *other* parts change, and suddenly whenever any major transitions are experienced (like leaving school, falling in or out of love, or becoming a parent). What may happen is that whenever a major change occurs in the social relationships by which we define ourselves, it calls into question the reliability of the form book or manual we use to predict what is going to happen next and what we ourselves are going to do or feel.

Reactions to loss of identity

As you are now, you know—more or less—what you are going to do next. You know how you are going to feel in the next few hours about the justices and injustices of the world, about love and death, friends and enemies, family and patients. But suppose one of your *us's* is removed in the next few moments as you are reading this (suppose a colleague died or a friend betrayed you) how sure could you be that the new, reduced *you* would go on acting and feeling the same way? The greater the chunk of *us* that gets cut off, the less can *I* predict how the *me* that is left will behave, so the more *I* become a puzzle to myself—chunks like the deaths of a friend or a parent, the loss of a job, perhaps even the loss of 'cool', certainly the loss of linguistic skill.

The immediate natural response to the loss of an important part of *me* is often a great sense of confusion. If I am no longer what I was, what on earth am I now? Perhaps I am now utterly different; just the opposite to what I was. If I was strong, am I now weak? If I felt constrained, am I now free? If I was always pushed to one side, can I now be a burden? One solution to the confusion of a major loss is to construe myself as utterly helpless: since I can do nothing to predict what it is best to do, it is best to do nothing but simply trust myself to the waves or the arms that hold me, however rough or restrictive. Such a strategy may provide a useful, perhaps essential, resting place. The more conventional responses to loss, anger and sadness, may have to wait to emerge until the person inside has sorted him or herself out enough to begin to estimate the size of the loss, to finger the edges of the wound. Acceptance of the way things really are now probably has to wait until the person has worked out a new personal technology, that is, a new way of guessing accurately what he or she will do and feel next.

This process of working out the new form book takes time, courage and skilled experimentation. Powerful emotions of fear, love, grief and revenge may emerge. Where the loss was great and where it takes many months or years to audit the full extent of the loss (like recovery from brain injury), people may fight very hard to deny the changes that the rest of us see. Sometimes they hold on to a crippled identity despite the recovery we can see. Sometimes people lose their strength and sink into the sick role forever or kill themselves. Much depends not only on the help they get but also on the sort of person they have always been. Some people feel safe only if they can foresee the future weeks ahead; others enjoy poking and prodding the world all the time just to see what will happen; some have learnt never to trust another; some have never discovered how to trust themselves. Such personal styles will affect how helpless and anxious they feel.

Before turning to the losses experienced when a person becomes dysphasic it may be helpful to link the views expressed here with the work of Kubler-Ross (1970), Parkes (1975) and Bowlby (1980). These authors have variously and vividly described 'stages' and 'processes' which bereaved people characteristically experience. The death of a loved one may leave the bereaved person in a state of numb confusion at first, or they may deny it or rage against what has happened to them. Entangled with these feelings are intensely painful feelings of loss. This may be experienced both as the objectively real absence of the dead person and also as the destruction of a part of the bereaved person. Similarly the loss of a limb, or a job, or speech may be experienced not simply as an external loss apparent to everyone but also as a mutilation of the person's identity or even a contradiction of his or her self-definition.

The losses suffered by dysphasic people

This section will consider people who have become dysphasic and examine some of the losses they suffer and the new evidence about themselves that they have to come to terms with. Those who suffer any form of brain damage will lose their current roles in life by virtue of being ill. By becoming patients they can no longer behave in previously established ways. The person who suffers brain damage with dysphasia clearly loses like this, but is also marked in many other specific ways. To describe the dysphasic as suffering a 'loss of communicative skills' is a mere generalization and the complexities of the loss need to be highlighted.

The most obvious and acute loss is the inability to communicate everyday needs to nursing staff on a hospital ward. However, other difficulties seem to present themselves even in the early stages of illness which have perhaps more complex implications. One of the problems encountered by many dysphasics is with making straightforward enquiries to the medical staff in hospital. For most of us when in hospital, there is some opportunity to question what is happening to us while there and also a right to some explanation of the problem. Dysphasics can neither express themselves sufficiently to extract the information nor understand the information if it is voluntarily offered. This adds to the weight of dependency which the dyspasic has already been forced to carry.

There is also the problem of expressing anger in a conventional way. When people fail to understand your needs it is common to feel frustration and anger. However, dysphasic people may have to resort to gross nonverbal methods and emotional utterances to express it. This means their general behaviour is changed and others may well interpret it as a form of regression to childish or immature behaviour which the adult is expected to have outgrown. The patient who is thought to be regressed is often treated and managed differently from the patient with intact social and linguistic skills.

The personal relationships of the dysphasic may often become extremely vulnerable at this point because of the reduction of two-way communication (see Kinsella and Duffy 1978, and Müller and Code, chapter 8, for further discussion of these points). Even if there is a marked comprehension loss dysphasics can perceive the comforting intonation in their families' words, but they may be virtually unable to offer their families any words of support in return. This is very different from the person who is in hospital with a broken leg who can reassure the relatives about the degree of damage. Similarly, discussion in any sort of detail with the family is hazardous. Many therapists will recognize the plight of a spouse whose partner is dysphasic and who may be attempting to manage all the family affairs for the first time. The dysphasic cannot explain about wages and health insurance, nor how to pay the bills, organize the shopping and household routines.

To be able to tease and joke with someone in a comfortable way is an important dimension in a relationship. This sort of fluency is a very high-level ability and many dysphasics find this out of reach. Losing it may damage the quality of many relationships. The ability to say affectionate things to people the patient is close to may also be lost. Often families understand that this is now too difficult for the patient. Unfortunately, the logical understanding of the situation does little to protect those families from the feeling of hurt and loss.

In a more general sense, telephone calls which many patients in hospital now rely on are no source of joy to the dysphasic. They are either an impossibility or else fraught with difficulty and tension. Even when the patient returns home the telephone can take on the nightmarish qualities it already has for those people with fluency problems. Often a person who is bereaved or ill may receive tremendous comfort from cards and letters, but the dysphasic who has associated reading difficulties may find this source of support meaningless.

People frequently talk about 'crossed wires' in their dealings with normal speakers and how this can affect a relationship. This is obviously greatly aggravated by being dysphasic and thus the subtler shades of relating to someone else have been blotted out, left in the dark at a time when someone is being forced to make a major reorganization of a whole life. The extent of this loss is so vast that it is easy to see how a large part of the self can be swept away by dysphasia. Some of the personal reports from recovered dysphasics offer a helpful impression of how it feels to become dysphasic. Wulf (1973) offered a powerful description of the predicament when she titled her book 'Aphasia, my world alone'. Hodgins (1968) also describes the despair he felt when he experienced what he described as his tongue's 'new and unwelcome capacity'.

The changing combinations of emotions that slide about as the dysphasic struggles to cope with his difficulties are a central issue for the therapist to deal with. The recognition of this grieving process is emphasized by Tanner (1980) who also noted the problems associated with aphasia such as the loss of home through institutionalization, loss of mobility through hemiplegia, and visual deficit. Bowlby (1980) also refers to the importance of the process of grief if a person is eventually to recover and adjust. He notes that 'this redefinition of self and situation is as painful as it is crucial, if only because it means relinquishing finally all hope that the lost person can be recovered and the old situation re-established. Yet until redefinition is achieved no plans for the future can be made.' (Bowlby 1980, 94). It may be useful to illustrate these points with the descriptions of the emotional reactions of two dysphasic patients.

Female aged 23. Middle cerebral artery aneurysm. Right hemiplegia. Aphasia with marked disorganization at syntactic level.

After neurosurgery this girl remained in a lot of pain and much of the attempted speech-therapy sessions were spent with her being in great distress and unable to concentrate. Four months later she was physically much better but still had marked dysphasia with a right hemiplegia. She was proving difficult for staff to work with and showed adolescent reactions to most things. Her family noted the same change in personality at home with a lot of facial expression when she was angry, pouting, shrugging her shoulders and giving up all attempts at communication. When the therapists attempted to explore any of these feelings with her she would react with a shrug implying 'it's not worth trying to talk about it'.

By the time a year had elapsed she had brought to the surface over-whelming feelings of frustration about her predicament. She began to try to question the therapist about whether she would remain in this handicapped state. She felt unable to make any social contacts and stayed at home except for rehabilitation arrangements.

At this point she began to raise the issue of her now being socially unacceptable, feeling that the normal relationships of her age group were now unattainable. She was also able to acknowledge the return of her sexual urges which served to highlight her present isolation.

During this period her mood appeared to fluctuate between manic behaviour and very deep depression. She was able to acknowledge the depression with the therapist and cry. On several occasions she gestured slitting her throat as an indication of her wish to die rather than remain in her present state. She was able to acknowledge this and attempted to talk about it with the therapist.

Although 18 months after the surgery there was little improvement physically and only a moderate amount in her speech, her mood and attitude did change. She became more emotionally robust and would demand independence from the staff at the rehabilitation centre, flirt with ambulance men and generally make social contacts.

This woman remains dysphasic and is likely to remain so for the rest of her life. However, a new person does seem to have emerged from the catastrophe, and although she remains very angry with life and more particularly with the neurosurgeon for damaging her in order to save her life, there is a new interest in people, her surroundings and her future.

Male aged 54, intracerebral haemorrhage. No paralysis.
Wernicke's aphasia.

The second patient was a professional man in his mid-fifties who depended on his verbal skills for his work. Initially he was extremely confused but was able to recognize the offer of help. After a month some relevant language did emerge and he showed some ability to understand, read and write at a very simple level.

However, the level of work remained very simple and this immediately brought into focus his feelings of anger about the injustice of what had happened to him. He felt great resentment at having to do the simple therapeutic tasks and also resentment at the therapist for drawing his attention to his difficulties. It showed how very difficult it was for him to accept his changed status and how very much he wanted to hold on to his original role. This was an issue which had to be acknowledged and discussed before speech therapy could continue.

Six months post-operatively, he was still struggling with his anger particularly towards the therapist because of the slowness of his recovery. By now the speech therapist was the only professional to remain involved with him and there was the conflict of needing the therapist's skills while at the same time not wanting to accept them. The feeling of dependence was not comfortable for him and he felt out of his own control.

After a year of therapy the patient showed good recovery but not sufficient for the sophisticated level he needed to function in his work. Emotionally he was beginning to face the reality of his situation and try to establish what was happening to him. He began to talk at length about his life before the incident and, as Parkes (1975) describes, he seemed to be searching for his old self.

Eighteen months after the incident the patient presented as a much stronger person. He was able to communicate more effectively with others, participate in social activities and attempt to do some part-time work. It seemed now that a new 'self' was emerging and this seemed to give the patient the strength to be able to acknowledge the dreadfulness of his experience. He described it so well himself by saying 'it's so hard trying to become a person again'.

A psychotherapeutic model

Clearly no two patients will share exactly the same losses and experiences in becoming dysphasic. Yet it would seem that there is sufficient common ground for speech therapists to be able to develop some strategies for giving these patients positive help in coming to terms with their fate.

Although words are the conventional form of communication in psychotherapy, what really seems to be the effective force is the personal caring relationship where the patient is receiving full attention from the therapist. It seems a helpful analogy to compare the negotiations between a therapist and a dysphasic to the caring activities of loving parents who manage to convey their care even to preverbal infants by word, by tone and by touch. Thus it seems important to acknowledge that even with the severely dysphasic person some communication of care and help can take place.

This model of psychotherapy as 'good parenting' needs fuller explication. How to be a 'good parent' is well described by Winnicott (1964; 1971) and summarized by Heard (1978) and Newson and Newson (1976). Perhaps the major component of this approach is a commitment between the parties. Neither child nor parent can run out on the other over a long period: each 'makes do' with what the other has to offer, and each 'puts up with' the other's good and bad behaviour (fatigue, irritability, anxieties, miseries and mess, as well as joy, frivolity, and success). But it is an asymmetric relationship in that the parent is responsible for the child, not vice versa, though the child has to come to recognize the realistic limitations of the parent's powers to protect and to 'contain'. The notion of 'containment' is important and complex including not merely the 'holding-the-line' against a child's attack but also the taking-in, keeping safe and making sense of the child's feelings before handing them back. Bion's (1962) complex discussion is usefully summarized by Mollon (1979).

The dual functions of the parental role to protect and to contain the child must be emphasized. A major part of 'looking after' a child is taken up with protection from danger and exploitation by others, feeding and comforting, reassuring and confirming the reality of the individual's experiences (both joyful and painful). However, parents also need to protect other people (including themselves) from damage by the child who has to learn that anger is no reason for smashing the neighbour's windows. So there is an element of 'containment'. There also has to be a more subtle personal sort of 'containment'. If the parents survive the magic of the child's wrath and despair and fear, it will demonstrate to the child that his or her feelings are not terrifyingly omnipotent. In a rather paradoxical way this relieves the child of magical responsibility for feelings by requiring acceptance of realistic responsibility for actions. So the parent acts as an intermediary between the child and the rest of the world, interpreting it and both protecting and confronting the child with the way it really is. It is this support of the child in the confrontation with reality that leads to growth and independence and safe separation. It is not a quick or easy process, but nature is on the side of independent survival. Parents are not necessary for survival as an adult although they usually persist internalized in the adult's memory and attitudes: sometimes for good, sometimes for ill. This characterization of psychotherapy as child-rearing has obvious parallels in any successful rehabilitation from serious illness.

However, the major difficulty when using this model to decide what to do in the practical situation lies in guessing how 'old' the 'child' is today. Obviously parents need to do different things for toddlers, school children and teenagers, but patients do not always make clear just how old they are feeling at the time they seek help. Part of the difficulty is resolved by recognizing that our earlier selves live on in us over the years: the 50-year-old still has within him some form of the memories, strategies and needs he had as a 5-year-old and as a 15-year-old and as a 25-year-old. If any of these needs were not adequately met at the time they may well persist long into later life. So when we speak to someone, we are addressing a whole set of layers of implications and needs. The practical problem then becomes one of monitoring the most urgent level of need in the patient. Most of the time people feel the need to be treated as independent sovereign individuals capable of making choices, but when feeling weak and distressed and confused such choices may become burdensome and there may be simply a need to be looked after. It may be useful for the therapist to start by feeding another almost universal need, the need to be understood. If the therapist can focus on meeting that need, then that understanding is likely to reveal what needs remain to be met later.

However, some difficulties may get in the way of reaching such understanding. Perhaps most of us are in two minds about whether or not it is a good thing to express our feelings. Although it is recognized that it is good both to 'get it off our chests' and to 'put up with things we can do nothing about', these are often seen as conflicting strategies. However, it may often be helpful to complain about the way the world is treating us (to express our feelings) not as a way of changing the *world* or persuading anyone else to help, but as a way of modifying the *feelings* and of getting someone else to understand how it feels. Often this release of intense emotion is described as 'breaking down' and it is seen as a sign of weakness, of loss of control, of imminent personal dissolution and hence guarded against by the patient and discouraged by the therapist. If, however, the 'breaking down' can be seen as a breaking down of the barriers between two people, a brave launching of a bid for understanding and negotiation, then the therapist at least may feel it is worth encouraging. Thus the release of emotion may become not a deterioration or a backsliding but a healing process. Useful discussion of catharsis as a helpful process can be found in Heron (1977). When a therapist helps patients to cry or rage about the state they are in, the therapist is not *creating* the upset, but merely allowing it expression and helping it to be accepted and healed. Indeed it is unlikely that patients will express such feelings in clear consciousness unless they feel safe with the therapist. If the therapist does not appear strong enough to 'contain' the distress, patients are not likely to risk sharing intimate pain unless driven to desperation by the intensity of it.

The therapist's needs

Of course, it is not comfortable to take these risks with a patient. Intense emotion such as sadness, fear, anger and even joy, cannot be observed, let alone shared, without resonating in the therapist, who is likely also to have worries about being open to the needs of patients. It may seem that recognizing a person's needs carries an obligation to meet them however unrealistic or inconvenient that might be. The unreasonableness of such a feeling does not reduce its power to upset the therapist.

Another source of discomfort for the therapist may be uncertainty about the nature of dependency. Faced with a patient who is severely isolated and distressed or with someone who has always had to snatch every passing morsel of care because it was so scarce, the therapist may feel overwhelmed by the greedy way in which the patient accepts the care and concern offered. If a therapist sees dependency as an addictive drug, the demands of the patient may be unnecessarily resisted and this may lead the patient to making the demands even more urgent because the supplies seem very scanty and the therapist miserly. However, if dependency is seen as a sort of normal satiable appetite, the therapist may be able to give care when it is needed in the comforting understanding that patients will stop wanting it when they have had enough, and that the persisting or recurrent needs of physically dependent and isolated people can often be met by families, friends, and speech clubs once they have learnt to accept themselves.

It does not seem that these are worries that conveniently go away with experience: therapists also have needs to be met. Unless they build their own network of support and puzzle out their own feelings with other helpful people they are likely to become stressed to the point of inefficiency. And to be helpful to the patient they have to succeed in surviving. As a word of comfort, in the authors' experience one does not become blunted to distress nor necessarily worn out by it. Instead a tolerance is developed for it in the same way a tolerance for exercise is developed. Even with regular exercise people still get out of breath when they stress themselves physically, but the recovery time is greatly reduced, and the experience itself may be exalting.

Practical suggestions

There are a great many books on psychotherapy, but Kopp (1972) Smail (1978) and Storr (1979) seem particularly useful therapeutic allies for clinicians ready to look at their work from a new standpoint.

Referring back to Kelly (1955), one vital need is for the patient to find structure and meaning in the confusion. As one step towards this, it is useful to make quite explicit the structure of the therapeutic sessions. That is to say, both the therapist and the dysphasic patient need to know how long the session will be so that both can pace it 'safely'; both need to know how frequent the sessions will be and what limits there might be as to how long work will continue together. The degree of privacy needs also to be explicit so that it is clear whether the conversation might be overheard. Both parties need to feel free from the risk of interruption by telephone or intruders, and the patient needs time at the end of the session to 'put his street clothes on again', so it is important to signal the end of the session a few minutes beforehand. Finally, on parting it needs to be agreed explicitly when both parties will meet again.

However, the major steps towards structure and meaning must be taken through the process of communication between two people. Here speech therapists can help by demonstrating that they can to some extent understand 'what it is like in there'. The speech therapist can do this by guessing what it feels like and expressing it in words and gestures, facial expression, touch and even tears, and leaving the patient time and space in which to acknowledge or correct the guesses. Therapists can explore with patients how they feel by using tentative statements like 'I wonder if it feels you are completely alone now'. Whatever way the patient responds establishes a fact, something the two can acknowledge about the patient's plight. In order not to risk telling patients how they *must* feel, it is important to express these guesses with tact and tentativeness.

In such intimate conversation people often respond to quite subtle implications of wording and intonation even if not fully aware of the cues. It is therefore important for therapists to keep a spare ear to tune in to exactly how they say what they do say. Bennett (1976) has drawn together several useful papers on these issues. Some forms of question may seriously constrain the replies the other person can make by being highly specific or obviously assuming what the answer is or by being unanswerable until their implications have been unscrambled; for example, 'Have you stopped interrogating your patient yet?' It is worth noticing the way the therapist asks the questions so that 'open' forms can be found to give the patient room to confide feelings and more 'closed' forms to elicit precise information. It is sometimes hard to find ways of phrasing questions openly enough, and it may be more helpful for therapists to check their guesses by using statements about their own states of mind ('I wonder if . . .'; 'I get the feeling that . . .'). This makes it easier for the patient to correct the guess, or agree, or even refuse the invitation to reply. A particularly useful form of words is simply to reflect what has just been said. This allows therapists to take their turns in the conversation, demonstrates that they have understood, and puts the ball back at the feet of the patient without directing or controlling the flow of thought. Sometimes a direct echoing of the last few words in this way will be enough to free the patient to go on and expand what has been said. This is particularly useful if the therapist is not yet quite clear what the patient is getting at, sometimes more 'summarizing' or 'interpretive' reflections may move things on more rapidly. A skilful summary of what has just been said, makes it clear that it has been understood and may not need to be said again. An inaccurate summary shows up the need for clearer explanation and invites it. Such a summary may simply crystallize the explicit meaning of what has been said, but sometimes it is important to interpret the poetic imagery of the patient and a summary that reaches into deeper meanings may show that it is safer to speak more freely or emphatically. It is important to recognize that ideas which seem risky to the patient are often first presented in a disguised or unemphatic form as if safely to test out the therapist's acceptance. If the therapist were to challenge the right to say such things it would be easier for the patient to deny responsibility for a message that had been hidden or muted. The therapist's ability to tune into the imagery will also be a convincing proof of being on the same wavelength. The art of reflecting can only be learnt through practice and diligent self-monitoring, but it is very impressive to discover how effective it is when another person uses it skilfully on us. Rogers (1951) well illustrates the subtlety of the process.

A word should be said here about *answering* questions. Patients often ask questions which seem to put the therapist 'on the spot'. This becomes less uncomfortable if the therapist can recognize that questions are sometimes only softened complaints or pleas for a topic to be put on the agenda rather than demands for information or action. Often it is best for the therapist to untangle the message by 'reflecting' it before attempting an answer although this risks the accusation of 'never answering a straight question'. It is surprising how seldom questions in such relationships turn out to be 'straight'.

Turning from these practical details to the aims of therapy, it is clear that a major part of the work is to help express and discharge pain. After sharing the distress, the therapist can offer, to those patients who have sufficient ability, opportunities for attaching more complex verbal labels to their feelings. This can help patients understand themselves more fully, as it may in any psychotherapeutic endeavour and is an important aspect of the parent's task of containment for the preverbal child.

Still later, the therapist can move from such 'containment' of the distress and confusion (making things manageable the way a parent does for an upset child) to gently questioning the assumptions the patient is making about being useless, helpless, too dependent to argue or be angry or make demands. This can often be done by just keeping cool when the patient risks a bit of a tantrum or an angry complaint. Sometimes, just asking a patient if that's the way it seems may imply that there is another way of looking at it. If the question can be asked, presumably the other person must be entertaining the idea that it might be different.

Often the therapist can challenge the patient's feeling of worthlessness by consistently showing concern, by consulting with the patient to discover present feelings and then respecting those feelings and not overriding them in a 'professional' or 'expert' way. The free flow of communication between therapist and patient can also offer the patient 'evidence' that it is still possible to communicate with another person.

Finally, to be there, reliably and regularly, during the worst moments confirms the patient's worth. This is living proof that there is at least one person who thinks the patient is worthwhile and who has survived the sharing of the distress and confusion. By allowing the patient to be dependent for a time, and by not running away from the emotion, the therapist can offer a structure in which the patient can build a new self. But to be 'reliably there', therapists must survive. To do that they must take time for themselves not only in training but in making regular use of the same processes of care and support they are training their patients to expect.

Acknowledgements
We are confident that most of the ideas expressed here came to us from colleagues, teachers and patients. Since they seeped into us over the years, we find it difficult to make appropriate attributions: nevertheless, we give thanks.

8

Interpersonal perceptions of psychosocial adjustment to aphasia

Dave J. Müller and Chris Code

Introduction

Currently, there is a growing interest in the emotional effects aphasic patients have on their relatives and close friends (Malone, Ptacek and Malone 1970; Artes and Hoops 1976; Bowling 1977; and Kinsella and Duffy 1978; 1979; 1980). This is of importance to therapists concerned with helping rehabilitate the aphasic patient. Satisfactory psychosocial adjustment is of great importance to both patients and to significant others in their lives, and therapists need to consider this when planning, implementing and evaluating treatment. The work of Taylor and Sarno (Taylor 1965; Sarno 1980a) has given particular emphasis to this need.

The studies undertaken by Malone *et al.* and by Artes and Hoops, illustrate not only the difficulties faced by families but the misunderstandings which often seem to arise. Artes and Hoops, for example, suggest that the wives of stroke victims often believe that their husbands have communication problems even in the absence of diagnosed aphasia. They also found changes at an interpersonal level. For instance, many wives reported that their husbands were now harder to get along with, that the wives viewed themselves as nervous or irritable and that there were resulting differences in their sex lives.

Kinsella and Duffy (1978; 1979) in their study of 79 patients and their spouses, report a high incidence of adjustment difficulties. It was found that marital relationships were characterized by problems of interpersonal communication, diminished sexual satisfaction and loss of partnership. Furthermore, spouses felt isolated, anxious and overprotective and, if female, were more susceptible to minor psychiatric disorders.

A number of studies have focused on interpersonal perception and have investigated how relatives and therapists perceive the aphasic patient's situation (Helmick, Watamori and Palmer 1976; Mulhall 1978; Flowers, Beukelman, Bottorf and Kelley 1979). The work of Helmick *et al.* and Flowers *et al.* suggests that spouses of aphasic patients view the patient's communication to be less impaired than it actually is. These conclusions were based on comparing test results administered by clinicians with the judgements of spouses. This suggests that spouses might be more optimistic than Artes and Hoops reported, but that this optimism may be founded on an unrealistic appraisal. Similar results were obtained by Kinsella and Duffy (1980).

However, Holland (1977) in discussing the study by Helmick *et al.*, argues that the spouse who is able to make use of contextual cues, might in fact be in a better position to assess the communicative ability of the aphasic patient. In reply, Helmick *et al.* (1977) stress that their data do indicate a discrepancy between spouses and clinicians in evaluating language. This is similar to one of the conclusions drawn by Cook (1979) in reviewing studies of interpersonal perception. Cook suggests that 'perceptions of other people are for the most part very inaccurate; this is as true of important decisions taken by trained experts as it is of the uninvolved observer' (p. 145). Given that so many opinions about other people turn out to be incorrect, Cook suggests that the most interesting question worthy of further reasearch is to see what happens when one person misperceives another.

Mulhall (1978) has considered the significance of some of the problems which arise from the interpersonal judgements of aphasic patients and their spouses. It appears that these judgements are of a cyclic nature and often magnify the difficulties both parties have in adjusting. For example, frustration in the patient might lead to anger in the spouse; this can then result in the patient becoming depressed which may elicit sympathy from the spouse; this in turn might result again in the patient becoming frustrated.

The foregoing review suggests that positive therapeutic applications might arise by focusing on the interpersonal perceptions between aphasic patients, their spouses and therapists. Hence the aim of this present study was to design a scale which could be used to elicit interpersonal judgements of psychosocial adjustment in aphasia. It was intended that this would not only help guide therapy, but that the very process of completing it would in itself be of value and become part of the therapeutic process. Accordingly, it was thought necessary to include the aphasic patient as well as clinicians, spouses and friends. In doing this it was felt that the Scale of Psychosocial Adjustment could become a useful therapeutic tool for less severe aphasic patients and for those who might be considered ready for discharge.

Procedure

It was intended that the scale should consist of items which experienced clinicians judged to be of importance in assessing psychosocial adjustment in aphasia. An initial list of 30 factors derived from clinical experience and previous research (especially that of Malone *et al.* 1970; and Artes and Hoops 1976) was drawn up. Included in this list were factors relating to the ability to form close relationships, to overcome feelings of self-pity, to accept the communicator's problems and other similar topics. This list was sent to 45 speech therapists with an interest in aphasia. They were asked to mark the 10 which they considered to be of the greatest importance and the 10 which they considered to have the least importance. It was emphasized that all the factors were important, but that it was necessary to make some evaluation of their relative significance.

Over 80 per cent of the lists were returned, but only 60 per cent of the therapists felt they were able to complete it as requested. Some found it impossible to select one item rather than another. However, from this information it was possible to produce a shorter list containing what appeared to be the 10 most important factors, although this was not intended to be definitive or prescriptive. The number of factors was restricted in order to aid administration. For simplicity, it was decided to ask each party involved, that is the therapist, the spouse or a friend and the patient to indicate whether they thought that each factor would get worse, stay the same, improve a little, or improve a lot (see Appendix I). Full details on how to administer the scale and a suggested means of representing this pictorially are included as Appendix II, but it is important to emphasize that the scale should be completed independently. If patients or others need help with the scale, therapists should ensure that they have already completed it in order to avoid any possible bias. By adopting this procedure it is possible to evaluate the interpersonal perceptions of the therapeutic process as it relates to any individual aphasic patient.

Analysis and scoring

As described in Appendix III, the simplest way of scoring the scale is to construct profiles. This represents the overall pattern of responses by each individual to every question, and gives some indication of whether or not their perceptions are congruent. A further analysis can be undertaken of each individual's unique set of responses, which may help therapists better understand the roles of those involved, including their own. Finally, the response made to each question can be examined, which may suggest specific areas of misunderstanding requiring further therapeutic consideration. This is why therapists might wish to include in the scale other factors of particular relevance to any individual aphasic patient's needs.

There is, however, a more detailed way of scoring the scale which gives a numerical indication of the degree of congruence. This is explained fully in Appendix III where it is referred to as a 'Perceptual Congruence Quotient' (PCQ). The purpose of this is to enable the degree of agreement or disagreement between the involved parties to be quantified. A simple additive technique would be misleading. For example, a therapist marking each question 'C' would score 30 (10×3) as would a patient marking the questions alternately 'A' and 'B' ($5 \times 4 + 5 \times 2$). Yet the response to each question is different and clearly indicates a quite high degree of incongruence. It should be noted though that simply totalling the scores does give some indication of how optimistic or pessimistic each involved party is.

These points can best be illustrated by two brief case studies. Case Study 1 is of J.E., a 60-year-old male anomic aphasic patient at 4 years post-onset. J.E. is an ex-solicitor and married with 4 children all under 14 years of age. He has excellent functional communicative abilities. His problems are minimal and concerned with high-level expression and comprehension. Therapy had concentrated on complex expressive and comprehensive tasks including reading and writing. As can be seen visually from Figure 8.1 there does appear to be considerable incongruence in the perceptions of each person. It is also clear from this that the therapist considers the patient has reached a plateau whereas the patient's wife is much more optimistic about further improvement. A number of specific questions would also appear to be of some importance taking into account the overall lack of agreement between the parties involved.

104 PSYCHOSOCIAL PERSPECTIVES

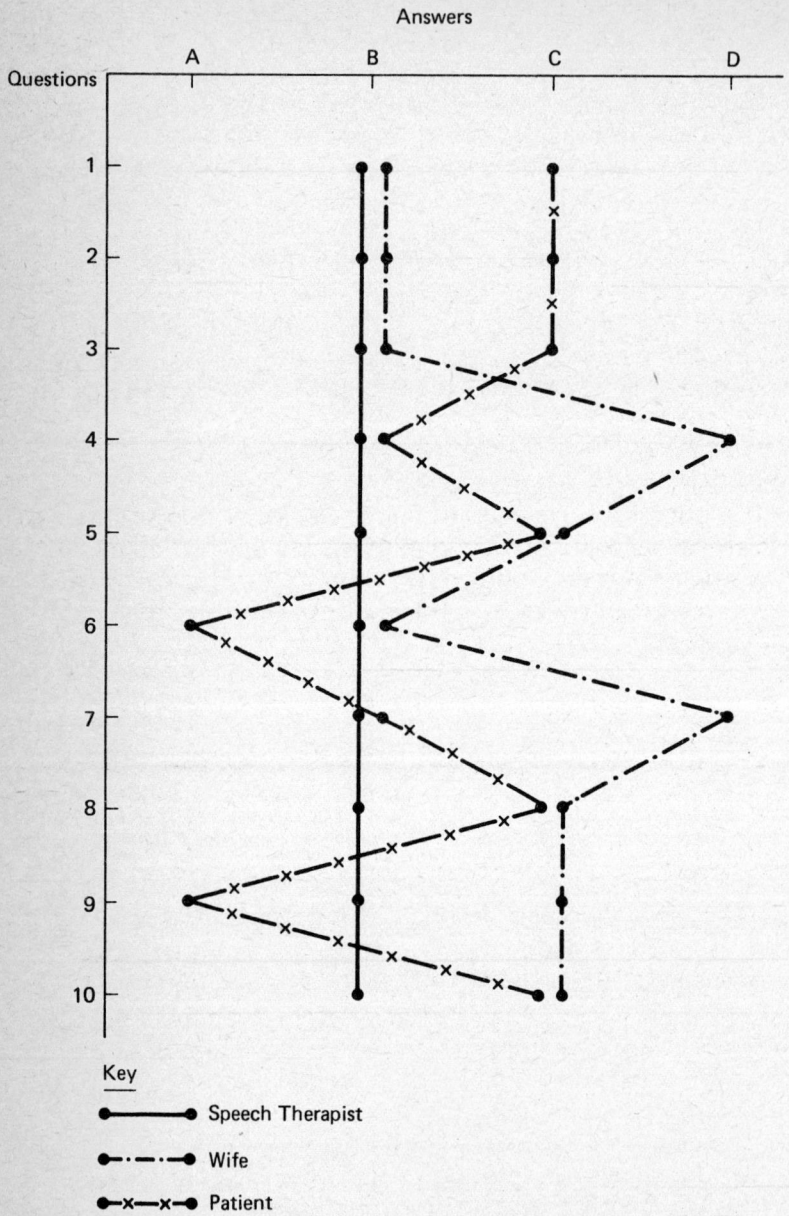

Figure 8.1 Psychosocial scale of adjustment profile for Case Study 1

Table 8.1 represents these differences numerically. In the far left-hand columns are the results of adding the scores together which produces a single measure of optimism. This confirms the initial impression that the wife is the more optimistic and the therapist relatively pessimistic, as reflected in a score of 28 compared to 20. Next to this are the calculations for the PCQ. For example, in answering Question 1 the wife and the therapist agree, but the patient disagrees with both of them. It can be seen from the total scores that the greatest incongruence is between the patient and his wife. By totalling the 3 incongruence scores together the PCQ can be worked out which in this case is 8.66 (26 ÷ 3). Finally, those questions which result in most incongruence can easily be identified by the totals in the final column. Hence Question 4 for example, may be suggestive of a topic requiring further consideration by the parties concerned, especially the wife.

Case Study 2 is of K.M., a 40-year-old male Wernicke's aphasic patient at 4 years post-onset. K.M. is an ex-clerical officer and a bachelor. He presents as being well adjusted and content. His functional communication is good and he leads a full and independent life. His problems are mainly concerned with comprehension. As can be seen from Figure 8.2 and Table 8.2, the interpersonal judgements are more congruent and certainly more optimistic than for the first case study. The brother is in fact extremely optimistic, but both the therapist and the patient score quite high. The PCQ in this case is 5.33 (16 ÷ 3). It should be noted that the therapist is the same in both case studies and that the scores reflect his differing perceptions of each patient. In the same way as in Case Study 1, this provides a wealth of therapeutic material for the involved parties.

Therapeutic implications

As noted earlier the scale is intended to be incorporated into the therapeutic process and should not be seen purely as an assessment tool. In fact, as an assessment tool it

Table 8.1: Psychosocial scale of adjustment profile scores for Case Study 1

Therapist	Spouse	Patient	Question	Patient v therapist	Patient v spouse	Therapist v spouse
2	2	3	1	1	1	0
2	2	3	2	1	1	0
2	2	3	3	1	1	0
2	4	2	4	0	2	2
2	3	3	5	1	0	1
2	2	1	6	1	1	0
2	4	2	7	0	2	2
2	3	3	8	1	0	1
2	3	1	9	1	2	1
2	3	3	10	1	0	1
20	28	24		8	10	8

106 PSYCHOSOCIAL PERSPECTIVES

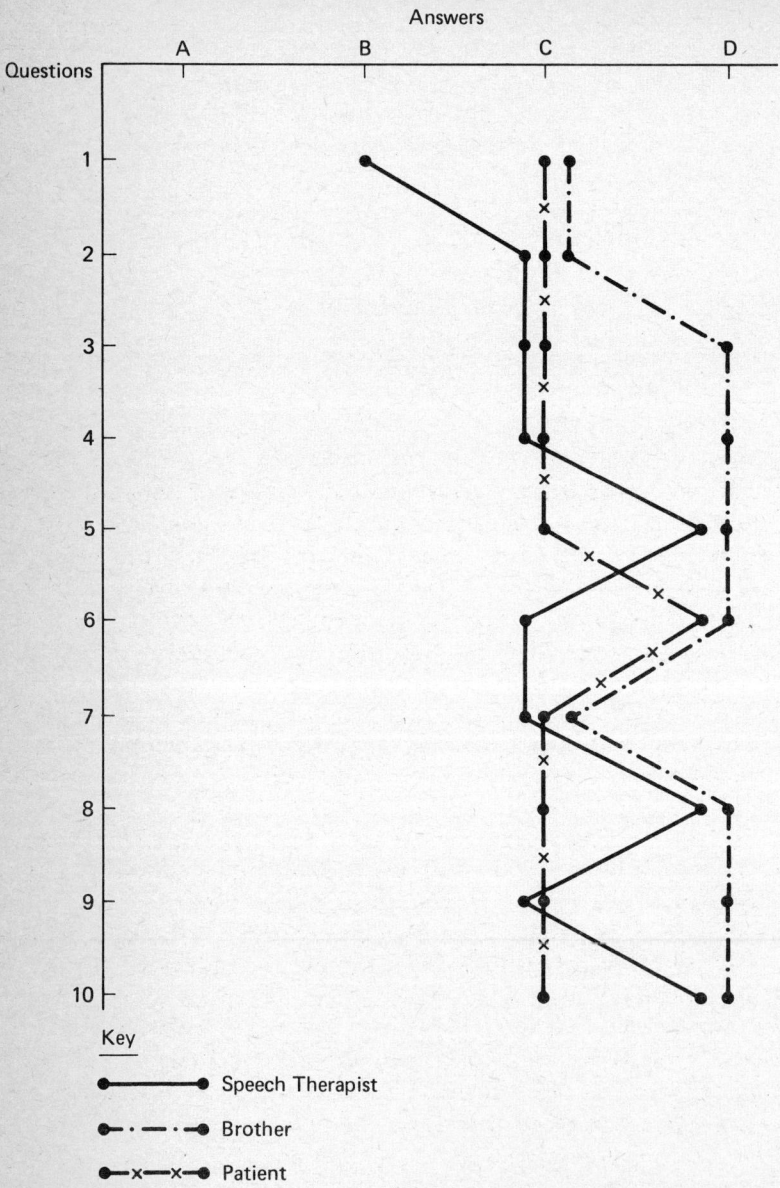

Figure 8.2 Psychosocial scale of adjustment profile for Case Study 2

Table 8.2: Psychosocial scale of adjustment profile scores for Case Study 2

Therapist	Brother	Patient	Questions	Patient v therapist	Patient v brother	Therapist v brother
2	3	3	1	1	0	1
3	3	3	2	0	0	0
3	4	3	3	0	1	1
3	4	3	4	0	1	1
4	4	3	5	1	1	0
3	4	4	6	1	0	1
3	3	3	7	0	0	0
4	4	3	8	1	1	0
3	4	3	9	0	1	1
4	4	3	10	1	1	0
32	37	31		5	6	5

may be misleading because there is no end point which is seen as necessarily beneficial, unlike many standardized measures of aphasia. The main purpose of the scale is to focus the attention of those involved on their experiences and perceptions of the patient's psychosocial adjustment. This, it is felt, is an enlightening process which helps those involved to understand themselves and others in relation to the situation. In this sense it can be seen as a therapeutic tool and as a means of putting into practice some of the ideas discussed by Brumfitt and Clarke (chapter 7, this volume).

At the same time the scale is indicative of the general direction that future therapy should take and may suggest whether or not there is a need for further counselling. It must not be assumed, however, that this is a one-way process in which the therapist is 'right' and can make therapeutic decisions for patients, spouses and others. In Case Study 1 for example, the therapist realized that his own judgement was unnecessarily pessimistic, perhaps because systematic therapy had stopped. Consequently, he revised his own judgements.

As already noted, the scale also shows the specific questions on which there is incongruence. Although in isolation these are not necessarily significant, they may require further consideration. In Case Study 2 a number of topics became the focus of discussion, particularly for the brother. This was also a reflection of his relatively optimistic viewpoint, which after discussion was not always found to be based upon sound enough evidence to change the judgements of the patient and the therapist. The topic which is often of utmost importance is how the involved parties feel about the effects of further speech therapy. This is particularly pertinent if the therapist is considering discharging the patient.

It should, however, be noted that the scale is not designed to enable therapists to decide on when to discharge their patients, nor is this considered desirable. This, it is suggested, should be the result of joint discussion between all the involved parties. Instead, it may be that on discharging a patient, therapists can use the scale as a means of making those involved aware of how they feel about the situation. In this way the use of the scale is exploratory rather than predictive. However, it might be suggested that therapists should be very cautious in discharging patients when there is marked incongruence which has not been explored by those involved.

Another important therapeutic aspect is that the procedure in administering the scale directs attention to the family, or to others who are significantly affected. As Sarno's work with the Functional Communication Profile (Taylor 1965; Sarno 1980a) has suggested, an important consideration is whether or not the benefits derived from therapy generalize to the patient's everyday environment. By involving other significant people, therapy can become a shared activity in which all the participants are able to develop a relevant role. In both the case studies already discussed, the roles of the wife and the brother were crucial in helping the aphasic patients construct a new lifestyle, one in which all those involved could take parts. This construction is important bearing in mind the findings of Mulhall (1978) referred to earlier.

A further value of the scale might be that it enables therapists to self-monitor their own perceptions of the situation. This makes it possible to compare what therapists think is happening to what other involved parties think is happening. The realization by the therapist in Case Study 1 that he was relatively pessimistic, changed his perceptions of the man and wife and he adopted a different perspective. It is clearly of prime importance that therapists evaluate their involvement periodically and not in isolation from others. Although subjective, the scale enables this to be undertaken systematically and empirically.

It is also interesting to speculate, as Cook (1979) has suggested, on the significant effects of misperceptions. The data collected to date are indicative that aphasia therapists tend to be relatively pessimistic compared to aphasic patients and their spouses. Spouses appear to be the more optimistic, although this needs further empirical confirmation. Thus, it would seem that in a number of cases the results of administering the scale demonstrate incongruity. This finding is in line with a number of the studies discussed earlier.

However, it may be that this incongruence is not an unhealthy sign. As Holland (1977) has noted, the spouses may in fact be correct in their assessments. Furthermore, it might well be that therapeutically, it is important for them to hold more optimistic views, in the same way that a cautious approach by therapists may be more conducive to a thorough evaluation of the extent to which the patient has recovered. Perhaps it should not be an aim to create congruence, as suggested in some approaches to therapy involving spouses (Bernstein 1979; Helmick and Marquardt 1979). In these studies the clinician took on the role of organizing the spouses to help them develop a more realistic appraisal of the situation. Further research to investigate whether a realistic appraisal of the situation as seen through the therapist's eyes, is in fact helpful, remains to be undertaken.

Finally, it is felt that the therapeutic potential of psychosocial approaches are as yet barely developed. In a very real sense aphasic patients have to negotiate a new understanding of their worlds and others in it. At the same time, spouses and friends have to learn to come to terms with a different situation. The psychosocial results of experiencing aphasia, whether directly or indirectly, clearly have significant effects. It is these effects which might provide the foundation for intervention and enable a more complete approach to aphasia therapy to be developed.

Appendix I: Code Müller scale of psychosocial adjustment

Please read the questions carefully and tick the most appropriate answer. Please answer every question.

---

1 Do you think the ability to work will:
   (A) get worse;   (B) stay the same;
   (C) improve a little;   (D) improve a lot.
2 Do you think with more speech therapy, speech skills will:
   (A) get worse;   (B) stay the same;
   (C) improve a little;   (D) improve a lot.
3 Do you think independence of others will:
   (A) get worse;   (B) stay the same;
   (C) improve a little;   (D) improve a lot.
4 Do you think the ability to meet friends socially will:
   (A) get worse;   (B) stay the same;
   (C) improve a little;   (D) improve a lot.
5 Do you think the ability to cope with depression due to the speech problem will:
   (A) get worse;   (B) stay the same;
   (C) improve a little;   (D) improve a lot.
6 Do you think the ability to follow interests and hobbies will:
   (A) get worse;   (B) stay the same;
   (C) improve a little;   (D) improve a lot.
7 Do you think the ability to speak to strangers will:
   (A) get worse;   (B) stay the same;
   (C) improve a little;   (D) improve a lot.
8 Do you think the ability to cope with frustration due to the speech problem will:
   (A) get worse;   (B) stay the same;
   (C) improve a little;   (D) improve a lot;
9 Do you think the ability to make new personal relationships will:
   (A) get worse;   (B) stay the same;
   (C) improve a little;   (D) improve a lot.
10 Do you think the ability to cope with embarrassment due to the speech problem will:
   (A) get worse;   (B) stay the same;
   (C) improve a little;   (D) improve a lot.

Appendix II: Code Müller scale of psychosocial adjustment guidelines for administration

The Code-Müller Scale is primarily designed to be completed by mild aphasic patients at any stage during their therapy programme. Separate copies should also be filled in by a 'significant other' (husband, wife, brother etc.) independent of consultation with the patient, and by the therapist before having prior knowledge of the results of the other two questionnaires. Where possible, a neutral therapist should administer the scale to the patient and, if necessary, the 'significant other' for maximum objectivity. The scale is designed to elicit information on the liklihood of the aphasic patient being able to adjust to changed circumstances.

It is realized that some patients may have difficulty in interpreting the response scale, and in grasping the meaning of the questions. It is suggested that therapists spend a little time on helping their patients interpret the response scale prior to introducing the questions. Figure 8.A1 shows a suggested method of explaining the response scale to patients who may have difficulty. It shows a hill with a human figure at point 'B' (stay the same). Below point 'B' on the hill is point 'A' (get worse, i.e. 'go down hill'), and above it point 'C' (improve a little), and 'D' (improve a lot).

Having introduced the response scale, the therapist should then proceed with asking the set questions. Therapists are recommended to give as much assistance as is necessary. This can take any form, from simply going over questions slowly, word by word to providing accompanying gestures, examples and so forth.

It may be noted that the rating scale can be seen as a series of choices (Figure 8.A2 is an illustration of this). 'B' (stay the same) can either be answered 'yes' or 'no'. If the answer is 'yes', 'B' will be ticked. If 'no', there is a choice between 'A' (get worse), and 'C'/'D' (improve). If the answer is improve there is then a choice between 'C' (improve a little) and 'D' (improve a lot). It is suggested that the starting point is always 'B'.

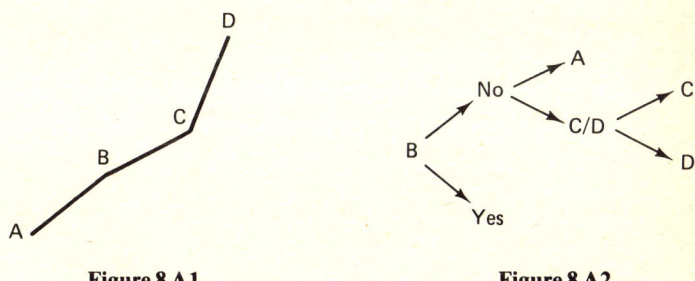

Figure 8 A1   Figure 8 A2

Appendix III: Code Müller scale of psychosocial adjustment analysis and scoring

1   The simplest way of scoring the scale is to construct profiles. This involves plotting the questions on a vertical scale and the responses on a horizontal scale and filling in each individual's response for each question. From this it is possible to draw a variety of inferences concerning (i) the overall pattern; (ii) each individual's set of responses; and (iii) the responses to each specific question. This is all that may be needed for therapy.

2 For research purposes it may be desirable to calculate a score representing the overall pattern. This has been termed a 'Perceptual Congruence Quoitent' (PCQ) and is calculated as follows.
   (i) Let D = 4, C = 3, B = 2, and A = 1.
   (ii) Compare the responses of each person to every other person question by question and record the numerical differences. For example, if on Question 1 the therapist marked D and the patient C, this gives a score of 1. If on Question 2 the patient marked D and the therapist C a further score of 1 is added, and so on until all 10 questions have been dealt with. The maximum incongruence score for any pair of individuals is consequently 30.
   (iii) Total the incongruence score for each pair of individuals involved. If 3 people fill the questionnaries in there are 3 pairs involved, or if 4 fill it in there are 6 (see below), and so on.

	Incongruence Score
e.g. Patient compared with Speech Therapist	5
" " " Friend (Miss X)	6
" " " (Miss Y)	7
Speech Therapist compared with Friend (Miss X)	6
" " " " (Miss Y)	8
e.g. Miss X compared with Miss Y	6

   (iv) Total the incongruence score and divide by the number of comparisons. In the above example the total is 38 × 6 = 6.33.

9

Group therapy: a learning situation
Margaret Fawcus

Introduction: the need for a more defined group role

During the past decade there has been a rapid growth in the setting up of dysphasic groups. In many cases they meet a real need, but they can also serve to mask the inadequacies of the service for the dysphasic adult. All too often patients with a real potential for progress, who want and need a carefully planned and structured programme, may find themselves in a group where they obtain general language stimulation on a once-weekly basis. This would not be such a serious situation if patients were also receiving additional treatment geared to their individual needs. Unfortunately this is often not the case, and many younger and well-motivated dysphasic patients must be content with very much less help than they need or deserve.

The literature evaluating group work is sparse and research into its efficacy almost non-existent. It is true to say that the full potential of group work has seldom been explored in any depth and, as Bloom (1962) observed, 'ordinarily group work reflects a dearth of clinicians rather than careful programme design' (p. 11). Groups supply social support, but there is a general assumption that they are incompatible with a progressive language programme. The group has therefore tended to become the preferred or recommended medium for dysphasic patients who are believed to have achieved their optimum level of recovery. Emphasis on the purely social value of such groups has given rise to the notion that they may, albeit with guidance and support from the professional speech therapist, be safely left in the hands of the volunteer (Meikle and Wechsler, chapter 10, this volume).

The rapid expansion of group provision has also tended to occur with insufficient definition of the role they are to play in the total management programme. It is essential to look more closely at the different types of group structures and functions. At one level there is the group for dysphasic patients and their relatives, of unlimited membership, which provides a supportive environment and the opportunity for relatives to discuss problems and share solutions. Professional help is usually available, and there may be a regular series of talks given by various members of the rehabilitation team. Such groups make no pretence to do more than provide social support and general advice and guidance, but they may obviously do this very well.

At another level, speech therapy may be given, normally on a weekly basis, to a group which may be large (up to 12 and even 15 patients) and in terms of type and severity of dysphasia far from homogeneous. This necessarily precludes anything other than a rather general approach to language re-education. Furthermore, the size of the group may give each individual member relatively few opportunities for active participation. Nonetheless, such groups do provide opportunities for social interaction and the potential for individual achievement. Much will depend on the expertise of the therapist since such heterogeneous groups make heavy demands on therapeutic skills. The exposure to such social stimulation would undoubtedly be more effective if it were more frequent, and if the groups were somewhat smaller.

This chapter is primarily concerned with small working groups (from 3 to 7 members) which can provide a structured approach to meet the individual needs of each group member. Furthermore, it will be suggested that such groups may be even more effective than individual treatment and certainly deserve much more of a central role in the rehabilitation programme. Far from being 'second best' provision for the patient who has reached a plateau in performance, it will be suggested that such groups might become a first-line and preferred method of treatment.

Social withdrawal and social reintegration

The group provides potentially one of the most effective antidotes to the serious social dilemma facing the majority of dysphasic patients. Havighurst (1968), in discussing the problems of senescence, suggested that the elderly person either withdraws from society, or that society withdraws from the elderly, and in some cases there is withdrawal on both sides. This situation is poignantly paralleled in the dysphasic adult. Patients may avoid making social contacts which serve only to reveal their linguistic inadequacy. In addition, hemiplegia may seriously limit their 'social mobility'. Friends (and even family) on their part may avoid social contact with patients because they are embarrassed or alarmed by the communication problems and by their own inability to deal with them.

The group, if it is functioning effectively, provides a permissive, supportive and yet stimulating environment which creates a need for speech and encourages communication, through whatever channel the patient is capable. Such an environment should create an atmosphere in which patients *want* to communicate, and where their efforts are not inhibited by fear of failure. As Whitehead (1973) reported: 'the relatives described with enthusiasm the change in attitude of the patients after joining the group. They had ceased to be depressed, now made more effort to communicate, and were prepared to venture into activities which they had hitherto avoided' (p. 7).

Brumfitt and Clarke (chapter 7, this volume) have discussed the rebuilding of personal identity. Given skilful management dysphasic patients may be able to establish roles within the group and so re-establish themselves as individual personalities in cases where their self-esteem has been undermined by the traumatic sequelae of brain damage. This is a very complex area of human interaction, and requires a therapist with a knowledge and understanding of group dynamics, social skills training and the role of nonverbal communication. The sensitive and experienced therapist can exploit individual abilities (and even eccentricities) which help to establish dysphasic patients as personalities in their own right such that even the more severe or global dysphasic patient can become a contributing member of the group. Indeed, Bloom (1962) claimed that the group programme was most effective with the most severely impaired, and even with those described as global at the onset of treatment. 'It is significant', he wrote, 'that many low-level patients were able to show marked improvement after little or no gain through individual therapy' (p. 15). Each patient has a much less passive role than in the more traditional patient/therapist relationship, which has important implications for transfer to 'real-life' situations.

The only valid criterion with which to judge the efficacy of any remedial therapy is by its carry-over into the patient's total environment. Lack of transfer is a problem facing all remedial workers and is wasteful of the time and expertise of the therapist. The good group situation, in providing so many and varied opportunities for communication, attempts to give the experience and confidence which facilitates transfer to home, work and the wider social environment. The small group work provides, as Whitehead (1973) notes, 'the medium for the practice of many social skills' (p. 21). Fawcus (1979) has further suggested that 'the dynamics of an accepting and yet stimulating group environment are probably even more important than the treatment techniques themselves (p. 16). Our own observations of groups confirm Bloom's view of their value in achieving 'an increased functional ability to communicate. . . .' (p. 12).

A structured language programme

One of the most obvious criticisms of group work is that it may fail to meet the precise needs of each group member and to allow for a structured approach to language rehabilitation. This may be true to a certain extent where the group is large and there is considerable disparity between the abilities of its members. In a smaller group, however, where the therapist can have an intimate knowledge of the performance level of each member in all language modalities (a knowledge which is facilitated by the greater time exposure the group allows) then treatment can undoubtedly be structured in such a way that it takes account of individual difficulties and the appropriate strategies to overcome them. If there is indeed any loss in the precision of treatment programming it is suggested that it is more than compensated for by other factors which facilitate learning.

Every task can be designed so that the stimulus elicits the optimum desired response from each patient. This means of course that the group members do not have to be absolutely matched for ability, although the more homogeneous the group in terms of the particular linguistic modality involved, the easier it will be to derive optimum benefit from each activity. The task (e.g. improving verbal comprehension or confrontation naming) may be the same for all members of the group; it is the presentation, and the type and level of response, which vary to meet individual needs and abilities. Such an approach demands great flexibility, and it must be made very clear that speech, gesture, writing and drawing are all acceptable responses, providing they facilitate communication between group members. This means that even the most severely impaired dysphasic patients may succeed at their own level. It is the therapist's role to provide the necessary stimulus to elicit the response in each case, to establish a series of goals and (with the help of the group and the patient) the various strategies through which they may be achieved.

Since the group shares the burden of communication, a two-hour session should not be too demanding or physically tiring for the dysphasic patient, although such an intensive approach is not strictly envisaged for the very elderly, frail or very confused patient. The social interaction (both verbal and nonverbal) of a successful group provides the necessary stimulus and interest to counteract boredom. In addition, an informal and permissive environment may reduce anxiety and tension, and therefore delay the onset of fatigue. There is little doubt that a group allows for a very varied and potentially interesting range of activities in all language modalities.

The group as a learning situation

What is it that the dysphasic patient has to learn? In one sense there is nothing new to teach, since the problem is now one of decoding and encoding the language that was once available. The patient may, however, be presented with a specific verbal task, such as confrontation naming of a series of familiar objects, which cannot usually be performed with any degree of success or reliability. With appropriate feedback and reinforcement this could be considered a simple verbal learning task. Secondly, and of much greater functional importance, strategies may be taught to facilitate the retrieval of language (encouraging, for example, the use of gesture to cue in a verbal response or writing down the first letter of a word). Thirdly, communication attempts may be reinforced, including the use of appropriate gestures and other nonverbal forms of communication. This can be in the form of incidental learning and it is in this area that the group may make its most significant contribution.

What then are the factors in successful group work which may lead to a higher level of verbal output and a greater degree of social competence and involvement? Any successful communicative interaction may be regarded as a learning situation if it reinforces the dysphasic patient's attempts to communicate and therefore encourages further attempts. In the absence of research data with dysphasic patients it is only possible at this stage to put forward some tentative ideas about the specific learning processes involved in the group situation.

Bloom (1962) was probably the first to discuss group therapy for dysphasic patients in terms of a learning theory model. He described it as a learning situation in which the individual's verbal behaviour affects the environment, producing a return effect with consequent reinforcement. Thus the dysphasic patient's behaviour 'is necessarily reinforced through the mediation of other persons' (p. 12). It is important to note that Bloom firmly placed the responsibility for such reinforcement upon all members of the group and not just the therapist. He claimed that group therapy resulted in a greater social effectiveness than individual work.

It can be claimed, of course, that the therapist working in the one-to-one situation can give equally effective reinforcement to the process of communication.

There is, however, an inevitable tendency to provide reinforcement in the form of verbal or nonverbal approval after almost every response the patient gives. This nonselective reinforcement gives less coherent feedback on performance and may even serve to reinforce the production of errors or inappropriate behaviour. The high level of predictability of the therapist's reinforcement can serve to reduce its overall effectiveness.

Early learning experiments showed that learning is more resistant to extinction if reinforcement schedules are random, and indeed once learned, 'the less frequently a response is reinforced the harder it is to extinguish' (Adams 1976, 26). This would suggest that the individual treatment session is *potentially* a less effective learning situation. In a group it can reasonably be anticipated that reinforcement, in whatever form it might occur, will tend to happen in a more random way. This is not necessarily the case, but in practice this does seem likely to occur because group members often communicate concurrently and not all attempts will fall on the listening ears or watching eyes of the other members of the group. In addition to this natural randomization of reinforcement, the very fact that a number of people respond appropriately to the dysphasic patient's communication attempt will be the most powerful reinforcer of all in establishing social and communicative behaviour.

The learning model can be taken still further by looking at the nature of the feedback provided by other members of the group. Another group member's inability to understand what a patient has said may indicate that the performance was not adequate. Should the therapist or another group member intervene with the appropriate model, detailed qualitative feedback on how the attempt differed from the target can be provided. If the patient's ability to monitor and thereby modify output is affected, then the provision of detailed knowledge of results becomes even more crucial.

Early experimental work into learning has amply demonstrated that knowledge of results (KR) facilitates learning and that, furthermore, quantitative KR leads to more rapid learning than qualitative information on performance. In other words, the more precise the KR, the more effective the learning process. In a group one might say that other dysphasic patients provide the qualitative feedback (by nods of understanding) leaving the therapist to quantify this information to improve further the patient's performance. Such KR can be seen as reinforcement, but it can also be viewed as a motivating element in the learning process.

Even more important, however, is the use of KR as essential information in a problem-solving situation. Adopting a cognitive view of learning (Adams 1976) then dysphasic group members can be seen as hypothesizing about the requirements of the situation, using KR to help them plan their next move. The group provides the ideal situation in which a patient can experiment in devising strategies and in working out solutions on the basis of feedback from other members of the group. Liberman and Teigen (1979) suggest that the 'accepting, cohesive climate in therapy groups also promotes symptomatic improvement and an atmosphere conducive to taking risks in trying out new problem-solving strategies' (p. 250).

The therapist's role is central here in providing sensitive quantitative and qualitative feedback whenever necessary. In word-retrieval activities for example, the therapist could score performance as follows: 6 for rapid and accurate response; 5 for delayed and accurate response; 4 for rapid but distorted response; 3 for delayed and distorted response; 2 for cued response; and 1 for attempted utterance. The quality of the therapist's relationship with the group is equally important. As Liberman and Teigen (1979) emphasize, while 'the technology of the behavioural clinician, based on empirical laws of learning, is important in treatment, the relationship with the group members also contributes to the outcome' (p. 267). They further suggest that therapists who do not have a positive alliance with the group do not possess reinforcing or modelling properties. In order to initiate changes in the group reinforcement contingencies, the therapist depends in part on a capacity to show empathy, warmth, and concern for those he is working with.

However, KR does not only give the dysphasic patient feedback on performance, but also provides an incentive to greater effort. As Welford (1968) notes, KR helps to maintain the level of arousal or activation, and higher levels of arousal are associated with more rapid learning. Motivation is not necessarily built in to the therapy programme, and language activities cannot always be intrinsically interesting. The addition of KR, however, would seem to be a very potent factor in sustaining interest, ensuring active cooperation and providing incentives to increased effort. The group itself, by providing an element of competition, also helps sustain the level of arousal providing the members are actively involved. It has been repeatedly observed that group performance actually improves under conditions of heightened stress and therefore greater levels of arousal. Whilst excessive anxiety and tension are obviously counter-productive, reasonable demands placed on a group seem to have a positive effect.

Conclusion

At present there are no data to support the claim that group work is potentially a more successful learning situation than the individual treatment session. Furthermore, there are many methodological problems to be encountered in carrying out research in this area. A possible solution would be a time-series study on a group (or indeed several groups) of patients, using the group members as their own control. This would require that the dysphasic patients involved in the research programme would all have been receiving weekly individual therapy equal to the amount of time they would receive in a group. It would also be essential that they had reached a plateau in their performance profiles for a period of at least three months prior to the onset of group treatment. This design avoids the problem of finding matched controls. The patients would then be admitted to a group at the same time, and performance could be reassessed at the completion of a six-month period. Any significant improvement could then be reasonably ascribed to the effect of the group environment. The one variable which would be difficult to control would be the quality of therapy which is dependent on the relationship between the therapist and group and the activities which are carried out.

It must be stressed at this point that it is not envisaged that group work should replace individual work in every case, but rather that small-group work deserves at least an equal status with individual treatment. There will always be patients with problems of such a severe and specific kind as to merit an intensive individual approach. However, the sheer economics of the situation preclude such an approach for the vast majority of dysphasic patients. Small-group work seems the only positive solution to the need for a significantly increased number of treatment hours.

It is suggested that the routine use of group treatment can more effectively meet the demand for intensive therapy for the dysphasic patient. Not only can the group successfully meet the patient's social and emotional needs, but in terms of learning theory, it may also offer a significantly better quality of therapy. It has been noted that group management demands a high level of expertise and understanding if it is to realize its full potential in meeting the social and linguistic needs of the dysphasic patient. There is an almost complete dearth of evidence to support these claims. The complexities of group therapy, and the many variables involved, make research a daunting task. This should not however, preclude a serious appraisal of the value of groups in the total speech rehabilitation programme.

10

The use of volunteers in the treatment of dysphasia following cerebro-vascular accident

Margaret S. Meikle and Enid Wechsler

Introduction

The use of volunteers in the treatment of communication disorders resulting from stroke has stimulated considerable discussion amongst aphasia therapists and others. There has been disquiet and uncertainty from some therapists who have felt their professional standing threatened and enthusiastic support from others who have welcomed the opportunity of additional assistance for patients. The personal experience gained by the authors while taking part in a comparative trial of volunteer and professional treatment of dysphasia following a stroke will be discussed. The subsequent local development of this kind of volunteer participation will also be described.

A comparative trial was carried out at University College Hospital, London between July 1976 and December 1978 and the results were published (Meikle, Wechsler, Tupper, Bennenson, Butler, Mulhall and Stern 1979). A research speech therapist was appointed who was responsible for all speech and language assessments and for directing the treatment given by the volunteers. The main aim of this trial was to examine the progress of dysphasic patients treated by conventional speech therapy from qualified speech therapists compared with a group assisted by non-professional volunteers who saw the patients in their own homes. It was found that the two forms of treatment provided essentially the same benefit although no firm conclusions could be drawn because of the size of the trial.

It was agreed at the outset of the trial to study a normal clinical caseload as far as was possible. Thus, all patients referred who, on test results, had a reasonable expectation of benefit from speech therapy were included. It was interesting to note that after sending approximately 1,000 letters to medical practitioners within the area, there was only a 1 per cent response. Information about the trial was sent to local hospital consultants and other speech therapists. The small number of subsequent referrals and even smaller number which proved suitable for inclusion was disappointing. The number of patients included in this trial, conducted in a densely populated urban area over a $2\frac{1}{2}$-year period, was less than epidemiological studies predict. This suggests that demographic details about catchment areas are necessary in estimating referral rates. Useful experience was gained regarding relationships between volunteer helpers and professionals and while problems were exposed, these proved to be soluble.

The role of volunteers

At the beginning of the trial a volunteer supervisor was appointed with responsibility for recruitment of the lay helpers. Helpers were found through an article in a local newspaper, by word of mouth and visits and talks to voluntary organizations. Most of the volunteers were housewives but there were also students, secretaries, postal workers and retired nursing staff. The patients came from more diverse social and occupational backgrounds. Attempts were made to recruit patients' spouses and other family members to the team of volunteers. It seemed, however, that the spouse preferred the freedom which a volunteer's visit allowed and many indicated that they were too emotionally involved to exert the discipline necessary to carry out therapeutic techniques. The initial response to the volunteer recruitment campaign was overwhelming, but because there was not a large number of patients immediately available several potential helpers withdrew. Throughout the project there were approximately 40 volunteers, several of whom assisted more than one patient.

The volunteers were interviewed for suitability in the presence of the hospital consultant who was in overall charge of the project. They attended a short introductory course given by the medical staff, psychologist and speech therapists. This course included explanations about the physical nature of stroke and a broad introduction to the types of communication disorders they might meet. Although the term 'stroke' is a layman's term and now widely used by both the general public and professionals concerned with the illness, it was interesting to note that initially some of our volunteers had no idea that a stroke was a cerebro-vascular accident causing damage to the brain.

When a patient was allocated to the volunteer side of the trial, the volunteer supervisor selected a team of three or four helpers so that a patient could receive not less than three and a maximum of four home visits per week. These patients also attended a group session run by the volunteers. The volunteers first visited the patient at home on a social basis. They then attended a discussion with the speech therapist involved in assessment to learn of their patient's specific communication disorder, and to be given the guidelines for treatment as indicated by the assessment results. These meetings with the speech therapist took place after each serial assessment to give feedback to the volunteers on their patient's progress and to develop the treatment plan.

Certain problems were experienced at these meetings between the volunteers and the speech therapist. The majority of volunteers had little or no knowledge of the types of communications disorders which often occur following a stroke. Speech therapists, through their training and experience, have developed a technical vocabulary to cover many of the descriptions of dysphasia. Terms such as 'Broca's dysphasia', 'perseveration' and 'articulatory dyspraxia' have meaning for professional workers in the field; however, even amongst professionals the descriptions of dysphasia are not universally accepted. Somehow the main elements of diagnosis and management had to be conveyed to lay helpers who had no knowledge of technical terms. This often proved to be a frustrating time for both the professionals and the volunteers.

An interesting part was the professionals' reinterpretation of the descriptive terms used in dysphasia to make them as clear as possible to the volunteers. It took much careful discussion before the main aspects of the disorder were conveyed to the volunteers and even after the problems were explained and understood it was necessary to specify which aspects of the dysphasia should be treated and ways in which treatment might be carried out. However, as the volunteers became more experienced, there was less frustration in what assessment results indicated for their patient. In the early stages of the trial the volunteers were concerned that, through their lack of experience with dysphasic patients, they might impede progress, and were anxious for support and guidance.

In order to make explanations as clear as possible to new recruits, examples and demonstrations were given. The volunteers watched films of a therapist working with a dysphasic showing the difficulties that the patient might have, for example in understanding short spoken commands and how, with built-up clues and perhaps the addition of the written label, the patient's verbal production might be facilitated. Stroke patients can feel distress at the way others speak about them in their presence and there is a tendency for some stroke victims to be erroneously regarded as mentally impaired. This can lead to great depression and frustration and the patient often needs considerable reassurance. Volunteers had to be prepared for such problems which can arise in approaching the dysphasic adult.

At the beginning of the project equipment was bought for the volunteers to use in their treatment sessions in the patient's homes. This included material similar to that found in most speech therapy clinics. However, the volunteers were also encouraged to use their ingenuity and initiative in the provision and use of their own materials, and these were found to be excellent. This was probably because they had time to develop equipment specifically related to their patient's own interests and environment.

As the project progressed a conflict arose between the patient's performance in a test situation at the hospital compared with performance in the more relaxed unpressurized atmosphere of home. It was found that some patients performed better under test conditions, while others did not do as well in these circumstances as their helpers felt was within their capabilities. This conflict could not be completely reconciled.

An area of difficulty for the research therapist was when the reassessment results indicated that the patient had reached maximum benefit from intensive therapy. Volunteers were often distressed by the realization that although their patient's dysphasia had reached a plateau, the individual still had a communication problem which was no longer responding to intensive treatment. The volunteers often needed considerable support and discussion to sustain them when they had entertained hopes of further improvement. Although therapy was discontinued, many of the volunteers continued to visit on a social basis, but less frequently, and the patients were still encouraged to attend group meetings once a week. The volunteers often became good friends with their patients, who tended to ask for help with personal and social problems. For example, some volunteers were asked to arrange visits to chiropodists, opticians, check on meals on wheels, report gas leaks or failing electricity. These are problems which professionals may encounter in the conventional clinical situation but which would usually be diverted to appropriate authorities.

From the professionals' point of view, much was learned from the volunteers about the patients' family interaction. It was felt that the volunteers played an important role in maintenance of the patient's relearned skills and social adjustment after discharge from intensive treatment although there was no objective measure of this. It was felt that the continued visits to the patients' homes and the patients' attendance at their social club encouraged communication.

At no time did this trial try to establish an alternative to conventional speech therapy. Ways of making the best use of professional skills and volunteer assistance to supplement conventional treatment were examined. It should be noted that 15 patients who were referred to the trial declined to participate and did so because of their reluctance to be seen by anyone other than a professional speech therapist. Although firm conclusions could not be drawn from the relatively small number of patients in this trial, the impression was gained that patients and their families, as well as helpers, received considerable satisfaction from participation. Good cooperation developed between professionals and the volunteers so that the question of volunteers threatening the professionals' role did not arise.

Implications

Since the publication of the results of the study outlined above, it has been suggested to the authors, by both speech-therapy colleagues and doctors, that it might have been unwise to report our findings. One of the reasons given has been that if it were assumed on the basis of this small study that volunteers could be used to replace professionals in assisting dysphasic people, this could hinder the necessary improvements in speech-therapy services for this group of patients. It is thus worth re-emphasizing that every patient in the trial had considerable contact with a professional therapist on the occassions of the serial assessments. The volunteers also visited the research therapist regularly and it was she who prescribed and monitored the treatment they gave. The indications were that the volunteers respected the professionals' judgement and advice and were anxious to follow this as closely as possible. It was not surprising to the therapists involved in the research that the volunteer-treated group progressed when such detailed advice was given.

Some previous reports of favourable outcome from volunteer assistance for dysphasic patients (e.g. Eaton Griffith 1975) have been based entirely on subjective impressions given by speech therapists, doctors and volunteers. In contrast the University College Hospital Study made no claims of improvements except where these were indicated by objective reassessment. It would, of course, have been possible to describe individuals on both sides of the trial whose morale appeared to benefit dramatically; however, what the study sought to discover was the effect on speech of providing volunteer assistance at home for those patients known to have potential for improving communicative abilities.

Aphasia therapists acknowledge the value of the help which a sympathetic relative or friend can give when able to work at home with the dysphasic patient. Although cooperation between speech therapists and relatives is particularly important when intensive therapy cannot be provided, many therapists consider it appropriate whatever the level of treatment. The research highlighted what therapists often find in practice however: that many families have great difficulty in giving this extra help in the home situation. Spouses of stroke patients are often elderly or infirm and some confess to being too impatient, while younger relatives may be unable to spare the time because of employment, household or other family commitments. It should also be remembered that dysphasic patients will sometimes reject help from close family or friends and there are others who do not have any relatives. In these circumstances it seems reasonable to suppose that, with professional guidance, volunteers can play a useful part in assisting the dysphasic person in much the same way as a willing relative or friend might do and it was in this way that the volunteers in the trial usually wished to be regarded.

It could not be concluded from the trial that all dysphasic patients are suitable for volunteer schemes. Patients were referred who proved to have psychiatric disorders such as dementia, schizophrenia and the associated problems, and alcoholism, and were not included because these disorders were felt likely to hinder the recovery from the dysphasia as well as pose problems for the visiting volunteers. Neither ought it to be assumed from the trial that any patient still recovering from dysphasia should be handed over entirely to volunteers. When considering patients for volunteer schemes, the speech therapist should usually take into account assessment results, the types of scheme available, patients' home circumstances and personality as well their own and their family's wishes in the matter. This will often be done in consultation with other members of the rehabilitation team, as home visits have to be fitted into an existing programme of out-patient appointments. Advice from the social worker will also often be helpful in making the decision. It was found during the trial that, providing regular professional support was available, volunteers usually coped well even in difficult home situations. This indicated that anxieties expressed by professionals at the beginning of the research period, about how lay people might react when faced with some of the psychological problems associated with stroke illness, were largely unfounded.

Conclusion: planning a volunteer scheme

This study which indicates benefit to dysphasic patients from volunteer assistance, can be seen as having positive implications for the planning of speech-therapy services rather than as posing a threat. The practical difficulties involved in transporting patients to and from hospital for intensive therapy present regular organizational problems for clinicians. Difficult journeys, and the frequent delays and cancellations which occur unavoidably in the hospital transport service, can all prove frustrating and counter-productive to both patients and staff. These factors, as well as the outcome of the trial, convinced the speech therapists at UCH that it would be advantageous to continue to operate a volunteer scheme after the research had ended. The provision of home visits from volunteers for patients needing more intensive treatment than could sometimes be provided by the speech-therapy staff alone, was seen as a potential asset; especially for those with difficult ambulance journeys or in need of additional social support. It was envisaged that, with speech therapists and volunteers working as a team, both forms of assistance could be provided for these patients.

Schemes of this kind need considerable organization and at the close of the trial, funding for the research therapist and the volunteers organizer came to an end. It therefore became impractical in a busy department for the existing speech-therapy staff to take over recruiting, interviewing and advising volunteers. Arranging introductions and home visits, and giving regular information and guidance to volunteers about individual patients was also too time consuming. In order to continue the scheme it was essential to have the services of someone with a good knowledge of dysphasia and of speech therapy, someone who could continue to recruit volunteers and also to liaise between the therapists, volunteers and patients. As this would require a considerable commitment of time, it was considered unrealistic to expect it to be carried out in a voluntary capacity. Further financial support was essential, as although the local hospital and community voluntary help organizers supported the scheme in principle, they were unable to help with funding or the day-to-day running.

Some time elapsed after completion of the project before a grant was obtained from the Regional Health Authority under a scheme which encourages new approaches to health care. This provided funding for a one-year project to promote the development of lay helper participation in speech therapy for dysphasic patients. The scheme, though based at UCH and under the supervision of a consultant neurologist at that hospital, was planned to operate on an Area Health Authority basis with the support and cooperation of the Area Speech Therapist and colleagues at other hospitals and clinics. A hospital Voluntary Help Organizer, who was also a speech therapist, was appointed as volunteers organizer. A more flexible way of using volunteer assistance is possible in the new scheme than that laid down by the previous research protocol.

In the present scheme all assessments are carried out by the speech therapists responsible for individual patients at the different hospitals or clinics where they are receiving treatment, but these therapists do not usually meet the volunteers initially to give advice or guidance. This is mainly because of the practical difficulties involved in arranging for volunteers, many of whom are themselves working, to visit the hospitals at the same times as the patients. It is, therefore, the volunteers organizer who visits the referring therapist to observe a patient's treatment and discuss the requirements for additional help at home. The organizer later makes a home visit to the patient, as a means of becoming better acquainted and meeting the family before selecting a suitable volunteer. The volunteer is usually accompanied on the first home visit so that introductions can be made; this gives support to the volunteers and also provides a reassuring link for the patient with their speech-therapy department. As in the previous project, regular group meetings are arranged when volunteers and therapists can meet, and short talks on stroke illness and dysphasia are given. There is plentiful opportunity for questions and discussion and guidance can be given on specific problems when required.

This new scheme is providing further information and raising new questions regarding the ways in which volunteers can best be recruited and deployed to assist dysphasic people. Therapists are found to vary in the ways in which they wish to make use of volunteer assistance, and it is important to consider this in giving initial information to potential helpers. While research projects and trials involving use of volunteers may find temporary financial backing from charitable foundations and National Health Service funds, the problem remains of obtaining the financial support to establish more permanent schemes. If this support is to be forthcoming in the Health Service, these schemes must be shown to be beneficial to patients, satisfactory to therapists and volunteers and cost-effective. It is hoped that aphasia therapists will develop their own volunteer schemes resulting in substantial benefits to themselves and their patients.

Acknowledgements

The authors greatly appreciate the endless patience of Mrs I.W. Fraser for her secretarial services.

Specific Approaches for Specific Problems

Therapeutic methods for a number of specific problems which arise as a result of brain damage are presented in this section. Gielewski describes methods based on the work of Luria for the treatment of sensory aphasia and Huskins outlines an eclectic approach for the treatment of apraxia of speech associated with aphasia at different severity levels. Some problems of reading and writing are dealt with in the chapters by Godwin and Hatfield respectively. The method described by Godwin for the treatment of the syndrome of pure alexia may have relevance to the treatment of other forms of acquired alexia, and Hatfield's chapter presents an approach to agraphia based on an information-proccessing explanation of the patient's problem which utilizes the patient's retained graphic abilities.

11
Treatment of articulatory apraxia in aphasic patients
Susan Huskins

Introduction

The title of this chapter might equally well read: treatment of cortical dysarthria or of articulatory problems in Broca's aphasia (Broca's aphemia), in afferent and efferent motor aphasia, in aphasia with sensorimotor impairment and aphasia with persisting dysfluency. There are as many labels for the condition designated articulatory dyspraxia as there are schools of thought about its nature. Darley, Aronson and Brown (1975) found apraxia of speech to be a 'motor speech disorder', whereas others deny the separate existence of articulatory dyspraxia. Schuell talks of sensorimotor impairment and persisting dysfluency (Jenkins, Jiménez-Pabón, Shaw and Williams 1975) and Luria (1970) refers to afferent and efferent motor aphasia. It is not the intention of the author to explore the theoretical issues involved in these different schools of thought, or to champion a particular viewpoint. The descriptions of these patients by different authorities and the kinds of treatment suggested by them, have a great deal in common in spite of their theoretical differences, and it is these practical issues which are of interest here. A fuller discussion of the variable clinical picture encountered, and the importance of differential diagnosis, may be found in Huskins (1979).

Whether articulatory dyspraxia is regarded as a motor or sensory-motor disorder and whether it is believed that it occurs in isolation or is always accompanied by a degree of dysphasia, therapy is a sensori-motor process requiring stimulation, action or response from the patient and feedback. In addition, articulation therapy is often concurrent with or embedded in a language programme designed to deal with whatever degree of dysphasia is present. It is the aim of this chapter to present practical ideas for the treatment of apraxia in aphasic patients at all levels of severity, bearing in mind the everyday case load of the clinician.

Principles of treatment

Treatment must be based on a detailed case history and an accurate differential diagnosis. Firstly, it is necessary to differentiate between Broca's aphasia and other conditions affecting a patient's expressive abilities, for instance dysarthria, senility and psychosis. Secondly, it is necessary to identify all the components of a particular patient's communication disorder. Is it an isolated dysphasia, an isolated dyspraxia or a combination of both? If it is the latter, one must determine which aspect of the disorder predominates and the degree of severity of the different components.

Additional handicaps must be noted and taken into account when forming a prognosis and planning treatment. Such handicaps might include deafness or visual impairment, the presence of other forms of apraxia, e.g. buccofacial or ideomotor apraxia, memory disorder or intellectual handicap. The patient's age, general health, physical and mental state are all relevant to the prognosis as are such psychological factors as personality, degree of motivation and presence or absence of supportive relatives. The aetiology of the disorder is also relevant. For example, a patient who has suffered an isolated cerebro-vascular accident (CVA) and is improving physiologically, is far more likely to benefit from the lengthy treatment often needed than one who is at a high risk of further CVAs or whose physical condition and general health are poor.

Though mildly affected patients can make excellent progress, it has to be recognized that the prognosis for many of the more severely afflicted is limited. When describing Group 3 patients (aphasia with sensorimotor impairment; Jenkins *et al*. 1975) Schuell emphasizes that progress is often slow though gains continue to be made for several years and functional speech can be achieved. Rosenbek, Lemme, Ahearn, Harris and Wertz (1973, 471) also admit that therapy may be 'a painfully long, gruelling process'. It is therefore vital that both clinician and patient set themselves realistic goals.

In order to discuss detailed principles regarding appropriate treatment techniques, it is necessary to consider several categories of aphasia with articulatory dyspraxia. It is acknowledged that within the general pattern of impairment of the group suffering from Broca's aphasia, there is a great range of speech and language deficit, and widely differing degrees of severity of both the dysphasic and the dyspraxic elements of the disorder. These elements combine in different ratios in different patients and there is a continuum of breakdown from the grossest disorder through to the mildest. Thus any categories are bound to be artificial though useful to the clinician. Division on the basis of overall severity of the combined dysphasia and dyspraxia seems most appropriate. It is beyond the scope of this chapter to consider the wider management issues and broader therapeutic approaches needed to deal with the psychological, social and emotional problems which beset most of these patients and their families. Suffice it to say that the aphasia therapist must be aware of the importance of these factors, and include measures to deal with them, when planning a therapeutic programme. The treatment techniques to be described are only one aspect of this programme which should also include work on the patients' linguistic deficits.

Specific principles for the treatment of articulatory apraxia in aphasic patients

Gross disorder

Patients in this category are generally speechless and may be unable to communicate in any way. They are usually severely dysphasic and have apraxia of speech. This may be accompanied by severe buccofacial apraxia (causing inability to imitate oral and facial gestures) and ideomotor (limb) apraxia with consequent inability to use gesture. Such patients may have had a trial period of speech therapy with no improvement in oral communication. Their condition may be of long standing and consequently they may be extremely frustrated and demoralized. Any further treatment must have the aim of providing an alternative means of communication, however limited.

Visually based communication aids and systems may be of value to some patients. At the simplest level, these might be picture charts or personalized picture dictionaries. At a more complex level, a pictographic system might be appropriate. Such a system was devised at Birmingham Polytechnic (Cameron 1976) and used with one patient with promising results, but unfortunately trials on a larger group of patients were never completed. (See Rowley, chapter 15, this volume, for further discussion). An even more abstract system is Blissymbolics Communication and a full discussion of the use of Blissymbolics in aphasia therapy is provided by Bailey (chapter 16, this volume).

A more popular alternative at present is to teach a manual communication system to patients not restricted by severe ideomotor apraxia of the unparalysed arm. Skelly, Schinsky, Smith and Fust (1974) have used Amerind with oral apraxic patients and they developed a one-handed adaptation of this sign system specifically for use with hemiplegic patients. It was found that in addition to providing a means of communication, the use of Amerind actually facilitated oral speech production. Because Amerind is a simple sign system and not a sign language it is highly intelligible to untrained observers and the patient-user does not need to have a high degree of symbolic ability. Many of the signs resemble natural gestures. For example, to signal 'hungry' the person rubs his or her stomach. The Makaton Vocabulary, based on British Sign Language, is rather more abstract but it is now being used by some English therapists with these severely aphasic and apraxic patients. It was originally developed for use with the deaf mentally handicapped (Walker 1976). For further discussion of pantomime and gesture in aphasia, see Code and Müller (chapter 1).

It may not be easy to decide which type of alternative communication system to try with a patient. Success in these grossly afflicted patients is likely to be very limited so it is vitally important to select the most appropriate approach. The following case illustrations may give some guidance.

Ted was a 48-year-old businessman who suffered a massive CVA leaving him hemiplegic, aphasic and apraxic. When first seen he was unable to vocalize voluntarily and could not communicate in any way. He had a severe ideomotor apraxia of the left hand but did manage one or two spontaneous gestures as time went on. Attempts at direct work on speech gave rise to enormous frustration and extremely limited progress. After several weeks work he could produce /a/ and /m/ with much facilitation, but had great difficulty sequencing these sounds and a strong tendency to perseverate when new sounds were attempted. Reading and writing were severely limited by his aphasia and comprehension of speech was variable.

Ability to indicate 'yes' and 'no' appropriately was inconsistent. Ted demonstrated some ability to draw, so eventually an attempt was made to teach him an extremely simple pictographic communication system (Cameron 1976) using symbols to communicate everyday needs. He demonstrated some ability in this area but unfortunately died before any real progress was made.

A different approach was felt to be appropriate for Mr S, a 45-year-old Punjabi-speaking labourer. He suffered a severe CVA leaving him hemiplegic, dysphasic and virtually apraxic. Attempts at speech work were frustrated by his severe apraxia and the foreign-language barrier in addition to his dysphasia. He appeared to have some gestural ability so it was decided to include him in a small group of patients learning to use Makaton. His treatment continues at the time of writing but is hampered by irregular attendance.

Very severe disorder

These patients make virtually no spontaneous speech attempts though they may have some ability to imitate oral and buccofacial tasks. They are usually at least moderately dysphasic and often have a degree of ideomotor apraxia. Frustration may lead them to completely inhibit speech attempts but their disability is not of such long standing as the previous group. They may have severe oral apraxia making it difficult to cooperate with direct work on articulation in the early stages of recovery. It is tempting to regard work on speech output as too frustrating to be of any value and many therapists prefer to concentrate their own and their patient's efforts on language work aimed at improving any dysphasia present. However, in many cases it is worth attempting some articulation work, preferably for short periods but intensively. Such patients need a great deal of sensory stimulation and feedback to compensate for their frequently poor proprioceptive abilities and sometimes inadequate auditory monitoring.

This may take a variety of forms including the use of ice and of touch to help increase awareness of articulatory gestures and targets. An ice cube, or artist's brush dipped in ice-cold water, may be used to indicate which parts of which articulators need to come together. For example, tongue tip and alveolar ridge may be iced in this way to facilitate awareness of the desired target gesture. In addition, passive movement of the articulators may be necessary to guide the patient through appropriate movements of the articulators and sequences of articulatory gestures. Some therapists trained in the approach make use of proprioceptive neuromuscular facilitation, from which the techniques described have been derived. Luria (1970) advocated the use of automatic activities to help his afferent motor aphasics achieve the desired articulatory gestures. Examples of this would be; using the patient's ability to hum to elicit /m/, to yawn to elicit /a/, to sing along 'la la' to elicit /l/ and to blow out a match to elicit /p/. Feedback may be enhanced by the use of a mirror (though this is not always successful), articulatory diagrams (Figures 11.1 and 11.2), immediate audio playback and the encouragement of the therapist. Throughout, the therapist provides the patient with an audiovisual model by sitting where the therapist's face can be clearly seen and by

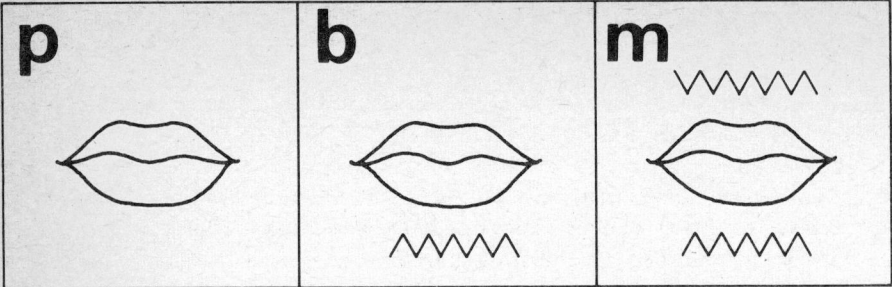

Figure 11.1 Articulatory Diagrams: The original diagrams were produced to the author's specifications in 1976 by J. Cameron. He designed two master sets which could be photocopied for use in speech therapy clinics by the author and her students. This ensured a plentiful supply of diagrams which could be used in a variety of ways with patients. The idea was based on Luria's Articulograms (Luria, 1970). These examples show how voicing and nasality were indicated.

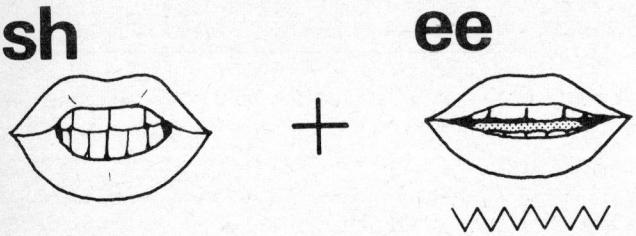

Figure 11.2 Articulatory Diagrams: This example shows how the diagrams could be combined to form simple consonant-vowel word patterns.

uttering the target very slowly and clearly (slow-motion speech). Rosenbek *et al.* (1973) describe an eight-step continuum using an integral stimulation approach (listen and watch me) which develops this technique for use with more able patients.

Any speech work attempted obviously needs to be in an appropriate linguistic context for that patient. Many patients find speech work so demanding that only a small part of each treatment sessions can be devoted to it. Also it must be remembered that only some of the patients in this category will make useful progress with speech. Encouragement of natural signing or teaching a modified manual system concurrent with work on speech output and the dysphasic element of the disorder, may help to alleviate some frustration.

An example of the kind of flexibility of approach needed is seen in the treatment of Mrs M, a 47-year-old housewife who suffered a CVA leaving her severely dysphasic and dyspraxic and hemiplegic. Her treatment continued regularly (once weekly with a supportive husband doing daily homework) over a period of two years, and included much work on speech comprehension and written language. At the end of that time she had a spoken vocabulary of some 50 words, a rather larger vocabulary of written words and about 20 Amerind signs, all intelligible to her husband. Initially, much work was carried out on articulation starting with imitation of voicing and production of isolated vowels and consonants. She found this difficult, but a variety of techniques were used to facilitate articulatory placement including mirror work (not very helpful), icing, articulatory diagrams, the 'listen and watch me' approach with much repetition, manipulation of her articulators, and the use of automatic activities. This led on to work on simple consonant-vowel (CV) and vowel-consonant (VC) combinations, building up the number of phonemes available and complexity of syllables and introducing real words at the earliest opportunity. She found articulation work particularly demanding and speech work often had to be abandoned for short periods and the emphasis directed to language work. After some time it was decided to provide another possible channel of communication by introducing Amerind. She mastered the basic signs quickly, in a form acceptable to her clinician and husband, in spite of a residual ideomotor apraxia of the left hand. At this point it was felt that she had obtained maximum benefit from regular individual speech therapy and arrangements were made for her to attend a supportive group.

Severe disorder

Here the patient's speech is severely limited and laboured and may be difficult to understand. There is often at least a moderate degree of dysphasia and usually hemiplegia. Although the prognosis for this group is generally better than for the previous two categories, some of the techniques already described may also be appropriate, at least initially, at this level.

The use of the 'listen and watch me' approach together with articulatory diagrams to visually reinforce articulatory gestures and movement patterns are certainly appropriate. However, there is much less need for sensory stimulation techniques such as icing, or direct manipulation of the articulators. Also, it is generally easier to elicit sounds from automatic activities. A variety of CV, VC and CVC combinations can be introduced systematically and in an appropriate linguistic context so that production of meaningful words occurs early. These patients are generally able to move on to more complex phonetic combinations (preferably always real words) and speech work can be reinforced with sequences of articulatory diagrams in association with the written word. It is essential that the therapist continually provides a 'slow-motion speech' model with much repetition—a precursor to the intensive controlled auditory stimulation (reauditorization) techniques used with higher-level patients (Jenkins *et al.* 1975). Much speech work can be carried out in association with language work appropriate to the degree of dysphasia present.

An example of this type of case is Mrs L, a 60-year-old woman who suffered a CVA a year prior to her referral to speech therapy. She was able to perform some items on the Minnesota Test for the Differential Diagnosis of Aphasia (Schuell 1965) and was classified as a severe Group III patient. Writing was severely limited but she had some speech. Language-stimulation techniques (e.g. sentence completion) were used successfully to elicit speech when it was not forthcoming spontaneously, but intelligibility was impaired by severe dyspraxia. Her treatment programme included much work on language in all modalities with particular encouragement of expressive speech. Schuell's reauditorization techniques and the 'listen and watch me' approach were used extensively to good effect, and the vocabulary and phonetic sequences covered were reinforced by the written form. On occasion, recourse was made to some of the techniques described previously to facilitate phonetic placement and initiate correct pronunciation. She made good progress over a period of approximately nine months. Staff at the home in which she lived reported that they found her more communicative and easier to understand.

Moderate disorder

Patients in this category will attempt to speak but their utterances are slow, laboured and often unintelligible. Some individuals in this group sound as though they have adopted a foreign accent. Others may be able to write better than they can speak but they usually have a degree of dysphasia, often apparent in all language modalities. The degree of accompanying dysphasia may be variable and more obvious in spoken and written language.

Reauditorization techniques are very appropriate for these patients, being a more challenging form of the 'listen and watch me' exercise. The treatment continuum described by Rosenbek *et al.* (1973), where the element of watching is gradually reduced and auditory stimulation becomes predominant, is of particular benefit. The patient's ability to make use of auditory cues means that treatment can be reinforced by the use of tape-recorded exercises or audio devices such as a language master. Articulation and language work may begin to come together more naturally.

J.F. is an example of this category of patient. This young graduate had a CVA following cardiac surgery at the age of 24, which initially left him severely dysphasic, dyspraxic and hemiplegic. He had had two years of speech therapy, initially intensive, before the writer came into contact with him. By this stage his disorder could be described as moderate dysphasia, with mild to moderate articulatory dyspraxia. He could communicate well in telegrammatic sentences, comprehension was good for everyday situations and speech was characterized by a 'shift in accent' so that he appeared to have a foreign (East European) accent. Speech therapy concentrated on improving written and spoken language structures, and articulatory agility and accuracy. The 'foreign accent' stemmed mainly from a tendency to palatalize alveolar and palato-alveolar consonants so considerable time was spent on the production of these sounds, especially /ʃ/ /tʃ/ and /s/. An oscilloscope was used to help reinforce correct production, in addition to auditory training to improve self-monitoring. A great deal of use was made of tape-recorded exercises aimed at improving language skills (especially in auditory and written modalities) and simultaneously increasing awareness of phonetic sequences (writing to dictation was useful here). Progress was made and maintained while therapy continued, but J.F. lacked the motivation to keep up this improvement once regular treatment ended.

Mild to moderate disorder

Patients in this group can communicate using speech but it is often slow and effortful. There is often prosodic disturbance and utterances are distorted. The degree of accompanying dysphasia is variable but may be only mild, and it is generally much easier to assess spoken language at this level. It is also possible to differentiate between dysphasic phonological impairment[1] and articulatory dyspraxia, both of which may be present and superimposed one on the other. The patient who is both dysphasic and dyspraxic benefits from language work as appropriate, and reauditorization techniques with some therapy aimed purely at improving articulation. This may take the form of drilling the patient on particular CVC patterns and consonant clusters first in monosyllabic, then in polysyllabic words. Those cases whose speech impairment is purely of a phonological type with no articulatory difficulty do not need work on articulatory gestures and movement patterns. They benefit from an emphasis on auditory discrimination, both inter and intrapersonal. In fact all aspects of reauditorization are relevant to improve self-monitoring, alleviate phonological confusion and improve sequencing ability.

A case which exemplifies all three aspects of this disorder (dysphasia, phonological disability and articulatory dyspraxia) is Mr D, a 61-year-old local-government worker who suffered a CVA. This left him with a mixed form of dysphasia and dyspraxia with speech containing both fluent and non-fluent characteristics. His articulatory dyspraxia was subtle but clearly demonstrable in phonetic and phonological analysis of his speech. He also produced dysphasic phonological errors where articulatory difficulty was not manifest. Comprehension was variable but he had some ability to communicate by writing single words spontaneously. His therapy programme included work on language in all modalities with much reauditorization and repetition work involving 'slow-motion speech' reinforced by the written sequence. Direct work on articulatory gestures was not appropriate but work on auditory discrimination and sequencing of phonemes in speech was seen as a priority. He made slow but steady improvement over a period of 18 months, after which time he communicated quite well using speech supplemented by writing.

Mild disorder

The patient's articulatory difficulties may be the most obvious element of the disorder though closer scrutiny may reveal a mild or even moderate degree of dysphasia and some dysphasic phonological impairment. Occasionally such patients present with an isolated articulatory dyspraxia though there is frequently a history of some dysphasia at an earlier stage of recovery. If the patient has any dysphasia, then any speech work must be incorporated with appropriate language

---

[1] The term dysphasic phonological impairment is being used to describe only those speech errors of a linguistic rather than an articulatory nature; i.e. fluent speech errors which obey the rules of English phonology, often referred to as 'literal paraphasias'. For further discussion of this point see Huskins (1979).

therapy. However if the articulatory dyspraxia is uncomplicated then articulation drills of gradually increasing complexity as described by Darley et al. (1975) are applicable.

An example of this category of patient was Mr B, a 75-year-old stonemason who suffered a mild CVA leaving him with a very subtle degree of dysphasia and non-fluent speech. He had a minimal word-finding difficulty which caused some hesitancy in expression and a tendency to use 'official' sounding vocabulary. However, there was considerable loss of fluency at an articulatory level with articulatory groping, in addition to the production of fluent phonological errors. His improvement post-CVA had been rapid but the speech disorder remained. Therapy involved high-level language work with much verbal description, reading aloud and encouragement of self-monitoring, as a means of improving articulation. He made steady progress and articulation was adequate provided he slowed his rate of speech but some of the dysfluency persisted and it was felt that this was unlikely to respond to further therapy.

Minimal disorder

These patients initially require great concentration to speak well and utterances may be slow and dysfluent. There may be a minimal degree of dysphasia. Treatment of the very mild dyspraxia includes the use of high-level articulatory drills concentrating on consonant clusters and polysyllabic words and incorporating these into 'tongue twisters'. There is much that patients in this group can do to help themselves. They should be encouraged to make use of a tape recorder to monitor their performance and to practice reading aloud and describing pictures and events or television programmes.

Mrs F.S. is an example of this type of patient. She was a 28-year-old teacher who suffered a CVA, leaving her initially with a moderate dysphasia, mild articulatory dyspraxia and mild hemiparesis, all of which improved rapidly. Treatment was carried out for a period of approximately four months with much high-level work initially on verbal and written comprehension and spoken and written language. Phonetic drills were carried out, systematically taking her through CVC monosyllables to consonant blends and polysyllabic words. She was encouraged to draw up her own lists for these drills, and to use a tape recorder for practice of drills and reading aloud. She was discharged from therapy six months after her CVA, with no observable problems though she was aware of being slower in speech and language skills than previously.

Conclusions

In the previous pages an attempt has been made to examine the range of treatment techniques available for therapy with aphasic patients with articulatory apraxia of varying severity.

Each patient has an individual deficit profile and unique therapeutic needs. A treatment programme can only be based on a full assessment of speech and language skills and a full case history including medical, social, emotional and family aspects. Eight categories of severity of dysphasia with dyspraxia have been considered. However, many patients will not fit exactly into these categories and thus their treatment programmes will need to be adapted accordingly. The case illustrations have been drawn from 10 years of experience with adult patients in various hospitals in England and there has only been space for the briefest profile of their speech problems, treatment and progress. The range of techniques discussed emphasizes the need for clinicians to be extremely flexible in their approach to these patients. Other aspects of the therapists work, not discussed here, include for example the role of counsellor, giving support to the patient and family, leading them towards realistic goals and providing contact with others with similar problems. Many long term cases benefit from regular 'stroke club' involvement, particularly when formal therapy has ended.

Suggestions for treatment techniques have been drawn from the work of Luria (1970), Schuell (Jenkins *et al*. 1975), Darley *et al*. (1975), Rosenbek *et al*. (1973), Skelly *et al*. (1974) and others, who have demonstrated their efficacy clinically. It is suggested that there is no one treatment schedule or formula which guarantees success with dyspraxic dysphasics but an eclectic approach is more likely to effect improvement.

12
Acoustic analysis and auditory retraining in the remediation of sensory aphasia
Elizabeth J. Gielewski

Introduction

The methods to be outlined in this chapter are based on Luria's (1973) definition of sensory aphasia and his clinical findings as to the characteristics of such a disorder. These methods have been used for the last 12 years at the Royal Talbot Hospital and have been judged to be extremely effective. Whilst it is always difficult to ascertain the amount of spontaneous recovery that has taken place it is felt that these techniques make a positive contribution towards recovery. Patients are presented at various times post-onset but generally in the range from six weeks to three months although there have been a few instances of patients presenting two years post-CVA.

Luria (1973) notes that

> in local lesions of the secondary zones of the left temporal lobe in man the ability to distinguish clearly between the sounds of speech is lost and the patient develops a phenomenon described by the term acoustic agnosia or, on the basis of the speech disturbance, by the more widely known term sensory aphasia. (p. 135)

An inability to distinguish between closely sounding phonemes inevitably leads to difficulty in the understanding of spoken speech. *Pat* sounds like *bat*, *pit* sounds like *pin* or *fit*. The patient is no longer able to grasp the meaning of what is being said because it sounds like a foreign language. The second result of such an impairment is that the patient has the same difficulty when naming objects or recalling words, some of which are severely defective in their phonemic structure, while the others are replaced by similar but inappropriate word—literal and verbal paraphrasias. The patient may also exhibit an associated writing disorder and find difficulty in distinguishing the necessary content of a word and confuse similarly sounding phonemes. Even the simplest words become impossible although motor stereotypes such as the patient's name remain intact.

Although the major studies by Blumstein, Baker and Goodglass (1977), and Basso, Casati and Vignolo (1977), suggest that a relationship does not exist between a phonemic hearing impairment (PHI) and severity of comprehension loss, clinical experience at the Royal Talbot Hospital shows that programmes based on Luria's hypothesis are very successful. In the paper by Blumstein *et al.* it was concluded that a PHI was not exclusive to Wernicke's aphasia and its severity did not correlate with the severity of comprehension loss. This evidence is used to discount Luria's hypothesis that 'the basic defect in temporal aphasia is the disturbance of auditory analysis and synthesis which leads to the loss of phonemic hearing, and as a secondary result, to the disturbance of all functions which are dependent upon this physiological function,' (Luria 1970, 127). However, Blumstein *et al.* use the term Wernicke's aphasia as a specific syndrome name whilst Luria's sensory aphasia is descriptive of a symptom (Luria 1963, 155), albeit an important one, that can accompany many aphasic syndromes. Therefore it is likely that sensory aphasia may occur in all the groups selected. The results in the paper show that a PHI was found to exist to some degree in all the patients included in the study; in fact a significant correlation was obtained between comprehension and a PHI, thus supporting Luria's hypothesis. However, the authors arrived at a non-significant result by excluding a group which appeared to have an anchoring effect—a procedure seeming to be statistically illogical. Basso *et al.* also obtained a significant correlation between a phoneme-identification defect and severity of comprehension loss as measured by the Token Test but corroborated the views of the Blumstein paper by rejecting this result for a variety of reasons.

Consequently, remediation of a comprehension loss accompanied by a PHI may be more successful when retraining programmes biased towards acoustic analysis and auditory training are employed. This paper deals with the assessment and therapeutic techniques involved in such a remediation programme for sensory aphasia and details an illustrative case study.

Assessment

If after formal testing the diagnosis of sensory aphasia has been made then the first step is to test for a phonemic hearing impairment. For this illustrated minimal-pair cards are used. The set of cards is made up as follows:
  (i) widely variant phonemes initially in words e.g. *wheat/seat*;
  (ii) phonemes whose articulation are visually similar e.g. *pen/men*; and
  (iii) phonemes that are acoustically similar e.g. *bin/pin*.
This is repeated with final phonemes including for example (i) *match/map*, (ii) *bell/bed*, (iii) *cap/cab*, and lastly with vowels for example *cat/cot*.

There are three stages employed in the testing of phonemic hearing. At each stage examples of each type of phonemic pair as shown above are included in the sample cards. In general, the severity of the patient's lesion will determine the number of minimal pair cards required. It is prudent to have a set of cards that covers every possible contrast.

Stage 1: The therapist presents paired picture cards and instructs the patient to point to the picture named. With each picture pair it is advisable to take more than one sample to ensure that the patient's acoustic traces are stable and discrimination is really intact. Many patients on the first presentation will achieve the correct response but when presented a second and third time become easily confused and uncertain of which picture has been named.

Stage 2: If the patient shows no difficulty at Stage 1 the therapist then presents him with cards containing three pictures. The patient is asked to point to one out of three pictures and if this is well within his capabilities two out of three. If the patient fails at either of these levels the therapist should draw attention to the manner in which the words are articulated and encourage the patient to notice the visual differences between the words. This is known as *visual clueing* and should be utilized to see if it facilitates success.

Stage 3: Cards containing four pictures are presented and the patient is asked to point to three out of four and four out of four pictures.

Patients with acoustic agnosia will have failed very early on. The patient with a more medial lesion will show intact discrimination at the one out of two and one out of three levels but begins failing at the two out of three and three out of three levels. The patient will also not be able to cope with any time decrement nor interference.

Therapeutic techniques

Acoustic analysis

If the patient fails at Stage 1 but can tell the difference between widely variant phonemes when looking at the therapist's mouth, then acoustic agnosia is the root of the comprehension deficit. The patient is then presented with something similar to the illustration in Figure 12.1 (i.e. words without the associated pictures) and taught to watch the visual signs—like a lipreader—to help discriminate the sounds. After going through the exercise the therapist asks the patient to point to the one said. Clinically, it has been found that patients at this stage often cannot maintain their attention for more than four paired words. Therapy is continued until the patient can visually discriminate acoustically and visually widely variant sounds.

When this has been achieved a few of the exercises are repeated but the patient is now asked to look at the words rather than the therapist's mouth. The patient is now discriminating through the auditory channel. If this is too difficult, the patient is asked to say the word to see if kinaesthetic information can help in recognition.

Once the patient can discriminate between acoustically widely variant phonemes the therapist moves on to those phonemes which may cause the most trouble. There are some phonemes which sound similar but are visually different (e.g. t/k, s/sh, f/s, f/th, m/n, d/g). Again these are taught using each clueing system in turn until the patient can distinguish between each pair using only auditory discrimination.

Next, those phoneme pairs which can only be discriminated auditorily, i.e. the voice/voiceless set are presented. Initially the difference between them may have to be exaggerated but once success has been achieved the amount of exaggeration is slowly decreased until the sounds are given normal emphasis. Once the patient can successfully discriminate between all phonemes in the initial position, the therapist can proceed immediately to the visually different but acoustically similar sounds, the most difficult being p/t, t/k and m/n. Again, each clueing method is utilized in the same manner outlined above. The voice/voiceless pairs are also covered. Work then begins on medial phonemes, e.g. *latter/ladder*. All voice/voiceless pairs are included and also p/t, t/k and m/n. When tackling vowel discrimination it is advisable to begin with vowels which are visually very different (Table 12.1).

ACOUSTIC ANALYSIS AND AUDITORY RETRAINING   141

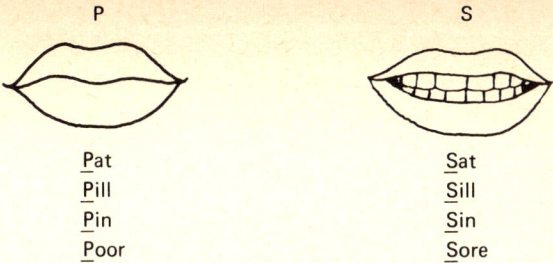

          P   S

        Pat   Sat
        Pill   Sill
        Pin   Sin
        Poor   Sore

Figure 12.1   Example of illustration to facilitate acoustic analysis

Finally, blends in initial, medial and final positions are covered. Discrimination between the ps/ts/ks blends occurring finally, e.g. *lips/lits/licks*, is often the most difficult.

Auditory training

With success at the final stage of acoustic analysis, phonemic hearing is intact at a single-segment level. Further training is required to extend this ability to discriminate two acoustically similar sounds and increase auditory memory to facilitate recall of longer speech sequences. This is initiated by presenting the patient with an illustration as in Figure 12.2. The three sounds are not acoustically similar so they should cause minimal difficulty. The patient points to 1 out of 3, 2 out of 3, and finally, 3 out of 3, and at this stage is allowed to look at the words. Following this, the task is repeated with the patient's eyes closed or the head turned so that neither the words nor the therapist's mouth can be seen. Again the retention task is built up to the 3 out of 3 level. The next step is to present the patient with three acoustically similar sounds, e.g. f/s/sh. The whole process is then repeated.

When the patient is completely successful at these tasks it is no longer necessary to supply the articulatory clue, i.e. the mouth drawings. Word lists can now be given where the patient is asked to recall 3 out of 4 words with eyes shut or averted.

Table 12.1   Examples of vowel triplets

sIt	sEt	sAt
bId	bEd	bAd
cAt	cUt	kIt
hAt	hUt	hIt
cOt	cUt	cURt
cOde	cORd	cOd

142   SPECIFIC APPROACHES FOR SPECIFIC PROBLEMS

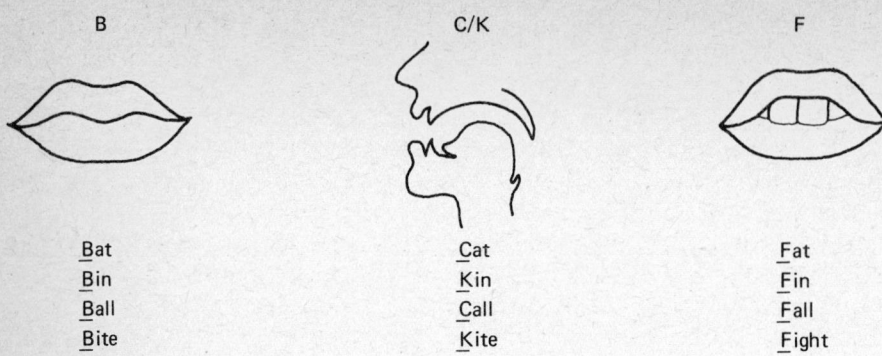

B	C/K	F
Bat	Cat	Fat
Bin	Kin	Fin
Ball	Call	Fall
Bite	Kite	Fight

Figure 12.2   Example of illustration to facilitate auditory training

Longer word lists are introduced as and when the patient's auditory memory improves. Examples of the types of lists are given in Table 12.2. Auditory retention is approaching normal limits when the patient is able to point to 4 out of 7 words without using visual clues.

Tasks to reinforce acoustic analysis and auditory training

A patient with a PHI tends to have a short attention span, is easily fatigued and cannot cope with minimal-pair training for half an hour. Therefore to consolidate acoustic training the following tasks are often used. Rhyming words can be dictated to the patient (five are usually sufficient). If the patient finds writing the whole word difficult the written vowel and final consonant can be supplied with the patient filling in the initial letter. If the patient can read, sets of up to four rhyming words can be presented to be read aloud. The written word pins the patient down and enables verbal production to be monitored. Another task using rhyming words

Table 12.2   Examples of word lists for auditory training

Initial phoneme changing

Hall	Ball	Call	Wall	Fall	SMall	STall
Hum	Sum	Numb	Dumb	Rum	Gum	PLum
GRumble	Humble	Tumble	Jumble	Fumble	Rumble	STumble
DWelling	Telling	SPelling	SWelling	SHelling	SMelling	

Final phoneme changing

riDe	riPe	riCe	riSe	righT	
burN	burST	burNER	burDEN	burGLAR	burNING
gallOP	gallEY	gallANT	gallON	gallOWS	gallERY

Vowel changing

pAle	pIle	pIll	pEEl	pOOl	pOle
shOt	shOOt	shUt	shIRt	shORt	shOUt
sIt	sEt	sIght	sEAt	sORt	sAt

is to present the patient with four words (Table 12.3), three which rhyme and one which does not. The patient has to indicate the non-rhyming word. This exercise can be graded to include all levels of phonemic competence. With sensory aphasics who can read short sentences, rhyming words can be written at the top of the page and short sentences can be written leaving blanks underneath.

Concurrent with acoustic analysis training some basic auditory attention training can be introduced. Four pictures which are semantically and phonologically different, e.g. *dog*, *bed*, *pencil* and *hat*, are placed before the patient. The patient watches the therapist's mouth as one word is said and points to the picture. The therapist then moves on to 2, 3 and 4 out of 4. The visual clue can then be discontinued and the task repeated.

Pictures of objects which are semantically similar, e.g. four foods, or phonologically similar, e.g. *bell*, *ball*, *baby* and *bag* are presented. Once the patient can hold 3 out of 4 words in groups of semantic and phonological similarity the stage has been set for further auditory training work.

Illustrative case history

Medical history

The following case history is of a 45-year-old woman who presented at the Royal Talbot Hospital with sensory aphasia. Only the progress made in the first six weeks will be outlined in detail as this has the most relevance to the techniques described. The patient presented at the acute hospital unconscious and with a right-sided hemiplegia. The diagnosis was a left CVA following an overdose. Her conscious state improved after two days to reveal a severe expressive and receptive aphasia. She received speech therapy once consciousness was regained but her progress was minimal. Nearly six weeks later she was referred to The Royal Talbot Hospital and admitted. She was an in-patient and throughout attendance received one hour of speech therapy per day.

Initial assessment results

The Eisenson Aphasia Test (1954) results showed that the patient could comprehend neither auditory nor written material at sentence level. Expressive speech was

Table 12.3 Examples of rhyming/non-rhyming exercises

PAT	HAT	MAT	LONG
PAT	HAT	LOT	MAT
FIT	WIT	FIN	PIT
FOUR	MORE	TORE	TEAR
CAP	TAP	WRAP	CAB

jargon and she was unable to repeat digits and sentences without several presentations. She was able to write some letters and only single and double digits. Spelling of words was severely impaired and naming ability was poor. Arithmetic skills were only mildly impaired and she had no difficulty setting the clock. She refused to read the test passages.

Therapy and progress during the first six weeks

Week 1: Acoustic analysis work was initiated by presenting written minimal pairs consisting of /p/ versus all other widely variant phonemes gradually refining the variance. Sets of rhyming words were given to dictation and she was also asked to read them aloud. Auditory training work was begun by presenting her with three pictures which did not belong to the same semantic group nor begin with the same initial phoneme. The task was gradually loaded by increasing the amount of pictures presented or selecting pictures beginning with the same phoneme or belonging to the same semantic category. By the end of week 1 she no longer required the visual clueing system and was able to discriminate p/b, p/m, p/t, p/f, m/n, f/v, s/z, t/k, t/d, t/n and k/l in the initial position and p/k in the final position. The discrimination of s/sh was very difficult and the patient indicated it was impossible to hear any difference. She was now able to point to 3 out of 6 totally different pictures, 2 out of 4 phonologically similar and 2 out of 3 semantically similar pictures. Reading of rhyming words had improved and she could manage three groups of five rhyming words to dictation.

Week 2: The aim was for her to discriminate all phoneme pairs in the initial and final positions and to increase auditory attention in the areas of acoustic and semantic similarity. By the end of this week she was able to discriminate between all phoneme pairs in the initial position and voice/voiceless pairs in the final position except for k/g. She could also discriminate between t/k and f/s in the final position and th/f in both initial and final positions. When presented with the p/b/m and t/d/n triplet she was able to point to 2 out of 3 whilst looking at the words. Auditory attention was improving and she could point to 4 out of 6 phonologically similar and 3 out of 6 semantically similar pictures. Comprehension at sentence level was now good. Her comment at the end of the week was that things were starting to make sense, 'I can feel something going on in my head'.

Week 3: The aim was to tackle the discrimination of phonemes in the medial position, the discrimination of vowels and consonant blends in all positions, and to continue working on her auditory attention. By the end of week 3 she was able to discriminate between k/g in the final position, all medial pairs and all vowel pairs. The consonant blends were quickly attained except for ps/ts/ks. She was also able to point to 2 out of 3 vowel sets as shown in Table 12.1.

Week 4: The aim was to continue vowel discrimination by increasing the number of units from which to choose. By the end of the week, she was able to point to 3 out of 4 rhyming words unsighted (this meant that she was not looking at the material at the time of presentation); 2 out of 4 words with the final phoneme changing, unsighted (cart/card caused some difficulty); and 3 out of 4 vowels, sighted. She was able to take five-word sentences to dictation, select the non-rhyming word from lists of five and give six members of a semantic category when presented with the category name.

Week 5: The aim was to continue presenting 3 out of 4 phonemes until stability was apparent and to reinforce auditory memory and attention by dictating sentences of increasing length. Spelling, using lists of words containing all the written variations of vowels, was started and general language work continued. By the end of this week 3 out of 4 phonemes were still not stable due to fluctuating attention. She was responding to language work and spelling was improving rapidly.

Week 6: The aims were the same as the previous week. By the end of the sixth week 3 out of 4 phonemes were more stable. The patient no longer guessed responses and indicated when memory or attention lapses occurred. Spelling was very good and she now was ready to move onto bisyllabic words.

Therapy continued for the next five months dealing mainly with auditory attention and retention and language work. Auditory recall was never stable at the four-segment level due to her attention deficit.

Reassessment at three and a half months

The Eisenson Aphasia Test was readministered and the patient completed all sections faultlessly except for the mental arithmetic section. Comprehension of both auditory and written material was at the abstract narrative level. Spelling was good and she could take at least seven-word sentences to dictation. Speech in a normal conversational setting was fluent but this varied inversely with anxiety level and was to be her main residual impairment.

Conclusion

Acoustic analysis is tedious and it is only the success patients experience daily that stops them from being discouraged. The gains made in a session need to be constantly reinforced. For example, when new ground is covered in a morning session, this can be reinforced through revision in a second session. This constant reinforcement is necessary to facilitate learning and this can only be achieved successfully in an intensive setting.

Acknowledgements
I wish to express my great debt to Mrs Betty Hill from whom I learnt these techniques. Also I should like to thank Harry Gielewski for his professional help and for his constant positive attitude.

13

The treatment of pure alexia

Rowena Godwin

Introduction

Most speech therapists are familiar with reading disturbance as a component of a primary aphasic language deficit. Less commonly seen are formerly literate adults in whom a severe reading disability is the most prominent finding. Benson (1977) classifies three types on clinical and anatomical grounds: anterior, central and posterior. The anterior type, known as deep or phonemic dyslexia, results from a lesion of the left frontal cortex, and shows the specific language features associated with Broca's aphasia. Words may be recognized but not read aloud. Even in the absence of recognition real words may be distinguished from orthographically lawful nonsense words, which suggests that primary visual processing is intact. The central type, alexia with agraphia, is due to lesions in the left tempero-parietal region involving the angular gyrus. Some fluent aphasia is usual, but the radical disturbance of phoneme, grapheme and word meaning is manifested chiefly in reading and writing.

The posterior type, pure alexia, is the subject of this chapter. It features an isolated inability to read and is known as pure word-blindness, subcortical alexia, visual alexia, agnostic alexia, and alexia without agraphia. The condition is commonly associated with a dual lesion of the left occipital lobe and the splenium of the corpus callosum, which are areas supplied by the left posterior cerebral artery; cases are also reported with lesions close to the angular gyrus (Greenblatt 1976).

Since it was first described in the nineteenth century, the syndrome has held a particular fascination for aphasiologists seeking to understand the neuroanatomical organization of language. Many explanations of the disorder have been proposed. Geschwind (1965) classifies it as an aphasic disconnection syndrome, due to interruption of the association fibres between the language area and the visuo-acoustic memory images of graphemes. It is also viewed as a form of visual agnosia which may have a basis in visual perceptual disturbances, including impairment of the ability to synthesize all the elements perceived into a meaningful whole. A primary eye-movement disorder has also been adduced. Comprehensive accounts of acquired reading disorders are found in studies by Hécaen and Kremin (1976) and Marshall and Newcombe (1977). Although there is disagreement over the nature of the underlying deficits, there is remarkable consistency in the accounts given of the condition.

Syndrome of pure alexia

In the immediate period post-onset there may be aphasia which can persist as mild word-finding disorder. Disturbances of colour-perception and colour-naming are common. An homonymous hemianopia is usual, although cases have been reported with intact visual fields. There is no gross eye-movement disorder nor impairment in visual acuity. The most striking feature is the selective loss of the ability to read, though words and letters are recognized when spelled aloud or traced onto a hand. Numerals and signs that function as ideographs may be spared. Spontaneous writing and writing to dictation show none of the errors in formulation and spelling which are characteristic of aphasic writing. Because of the inability to monitor visually during the act of writing, omissions and duplications of letters and syllables can occur. Handwriting is usually spaced out and badly organized on the page and copying is mechanical and laborious.

The disorder is classified by many authors into literal alexia, with inability to read letters; verbal alexia, in which letters are read but not words; and global alexia where no reading is possible. As there is uncertainty about whether these represent separate sub-groups, different degrees of impairment, or are the consequence of the particular reading strategy and the material used, reference to these categories will not be made. There being no paresis or sensory loss, the period of hospitalization is usually brief. This may account for the frequency of late referral for treatment.

Assessment

It is essential to distinguish this syndrome from other forms of acquired reading disorders, since the approach to treatment differs radically between these and pure alexia. Items from the Boston Diagnostic Aphasia Examination (Goodglass and Kaplan 1972) and the Minnesota Test for the Differential Diagnosis of Aphasia (Schuell 1965), together with careful questioning and observation, should be used to exclude a significant degree of aphasia. Care must be taken in the interpretation of any test involving colour. Comparison of the visual and graphic sections of one test battery with those of others provides qualitatively useful information, including the effects of print type and print size on performance. These should be supplemented by a detailed exploration of visuo-spatial skills, visual perception, orientation and letter-sound recognition, using selected material from the Standard Diagnostic Reading Tests (Daniels and Diack 1958), and Luria's Neuropsychological Investigation (Christensen 1974).

Where some reading is possible, distinct differences will be found between the pure alexic and the aphasic alexias in word attack and the pattern of errors. Typically the *aphasic* individual seems to recognize and retrieve words holistically and success is affected by such attributes as frequency and familiarity, concreteness, imagery, age of acquisition and the connotative meaning of the words. Semantic errors predominate, but errors also arise from visual confusions and from the influence of regressive and progressive assimilations from the surrounding text. The aphasic patient is unable to use phonological analysis or a spelling strategy to arrive at recognition, and experiences disassociation between the symbolic form of the written word and its referential meaning. Words seem alien and the patient will actively search the text for clues to unblock meaning.

In marked contrast, the *pure alexic* can decipher words by spelling them aloud. Difficulty is related to the length of the words, with errors tending to occur at the end. If the letter strings are correctly identified, then the meaning is readily accessible; however, where visual analysis is inadequate, the alexic is unable to scan ahead to use syntactic and semantic clues to clarify perception. Poor comprehension is mainly related to the slow speed of processing, though some defects of immediate memory can be present. Many alexics report a reduction in mental efficiency, particularly where there is reliance on visually and spatially based orientations; for example, recalling information on route maps, playing chess and expressing complex sequential relationships. If intellect and memory are markedly impaired and there is aphasia, reading rehabilitation will not be effective.

Prognosis

Evidence from many published case studies suggests that the prognosis for spontaneous and assisted recovery is poor. Some individuals are reported to have retrained themselves to 'read' by replacing the normal perception of letters with exaggerated tracing movements of the eyes, head and hand. Deciphering by spelling appears to be common.

Hinshelwood (cited by Gardner 1976), one of the earliest authorities on reading disorders, helped one patient to relearn the alphabet with six months of daily practice, and later taught him simple words from children's books. One highly intelligent 28-year-old (Ajax 1967) received intensive help from his wife, who recorded passages which he simultaneously listened to while scanning the text. Two years later he had made insignificant gains from his three months post-onset reading rate of 25 to 30 words per minute. The normal reader will process upwards of 300 words per minute.

Treatment: principles and procedures

This section describes an empirically based approach to remediation which has been used with a small number of patients. Its rationale is that by careful manipulation of the visual distinctiveness of the typography and the visuo-semantic characteristics of the texts, it is possible to develop a range of strategies to re-establish the reading process. Visual distinctiveness refers to the following:

Size of print

The clinical observation that large print facilitates reading performance finds support in the study by Woods and Pöppel (1974). They showed that both accuracy and speed of recognition improved markedly in an alexic subject as print size increased from 10 point (pt.) through to 48 pt. type. No such effects were found in normal subjects or in subjects with right visual-field defects. (It is interesting to note that 14 pt. is the recommended size for children beginning to read, and that larger print does not improve reading performance.) Minimum type sizes are recommended for each stage of the programme.

Density

Bold and medium print is more distinctive than light print. Patients often report greater difficulty with blurred copy or a badly lit page.

Typeface

Publishers and advertisers recognize and exploit the effects on the reader of different styles of typeface. The clinician must consider these differences in judging the legibility of printed material. However, it is essential that lower-case letters be used except where normal orthography requires upper-case. Individual upper-case letters may be more easily distinguished, but when they are grouped in words the distinctive shapes of the words are lost and a letter-by-letter analysis promoted. Handwriting, which produces special problems of interpretation is introduced late in the programme.

Spacing

The amount of space between letters and words and in the design layout appears to influence ease of recognition. Print should not be crowded and clear routes should be left for the eye to pass along the lines.

Similarities

Similarities between letters and similarities of word shape interact with visual sequential problems, leading to many of the delays and errors in identification. Common confusions are:

```
e   a   s   c   o      n   u   m   w      b   p   d      h   f   l   t   k   i
was : saw              from : form        for : off
```

Pure alexia is viewed here as a disorder of visual processing, with higher-order cognitive and linguistic abilities essentially unimpaired. Nevertheless, the linguistic demands of the text should be carefully controlled. Short familiar words are presented before longer and less common words; single-word recognition span precedes recognition span at phrase level; simple sentences precede compound and complex sentences following the principles which govern intervention for developmental language delay.

There is evidence that the normal literate adult is able to gain access to the internal lexicon (the knowledge each reader has of the meaning, the pronunciation, and the spelling of words) by various routes (Coltheart 1978; Spoehr 1978). These are predominantly phonemic, visual and articulatory, although both the alexic and the blind individual can resort to tactile and kinesthetic routes. Additionally, it is known that written words are recognized by many cues. These include: general shape and length; initial and final letters; and the presence of distinctive clusters of consonants, together with linguistic and contextual clues. Since it is not possible to know in any detail how the formerly skilled reader was able to extract meaning from print, or by what strategies and processes the skill was achieved, the approach described below assumes that the alexic patient will have tacit knowledge which can be exploited in rehabilitation. It is the therapist's function to tap this knowledge systematically, and to structure the material and the tasks so that the patient can progress with minimum frustration and failure.

Four stages are described below. The first two are concerned with letter and word discrimination and introduce phonic and eye-scanning strategies to deal with short, visually distinctive units. The third stage is concerned with material of increasing visual complexity, and requires both recognition and reading aloud. Not until the fourth stage is reading for meaning expected, in which memory processes interact with word recognition so that the propositional structure of the text is understood and interpreted.

Stage I

Stage I involves: upper and lower-case letter recognition (pointing); single words less than 7 letters; left to right search.

Step 1: When assessment shows gross impairment of letter recognition, preliminary work should include the tactile-kinesthetic methods advocated by Luria (1970). Large (circa 4 cm.) upper and lower-case letters are cut from black emery paper and pasted on cards. Beginning with the visually dissimilar letters O, A, E, and S, the patient traces round each outline with his finger several times, while the therapist describes its structure and shape and says the letter name. Substitution of these tactile movements by eye-tracing should *not* be encouraged as it is a slow and inefficient compensatory manoeuvre.

Step 2: When the two sets of alphabets are completed, practice matching and sorting tasks using a great number and variety of upper and lower-case letters cut from newspapers and magazines. This allows for generalization to different print types and sizes.

Step 3: Introduce flash-cards of short, visually distinctive words. Select these from a commercial range,[1] or print with dry transfer lettering (60 pt.).[2] A word is placed singly before the patient and named by the therapist. After 10 have been shown, they are presented in pairs, and the patient is required to point to one named by the

---

[1] The flash-cards originally used (300 Common Words: Kiddicraft) are no longer available. An alternative is Sets I and II of the small size flash-cards that accompany Ladybird Books 1a to 6b. Ladybird Books: Loughborough.

[2] Letraset: Letraset UK Ltd, 195–203 Waterloo Road, London SE1 8XJ. Helvetica medium is recommended.

therapist. Gradually the number of alternatives is increased. Whole-word recognition is accepted and encouraged at this stage, but the patient is *not* expected to read aloud.

Step 4: When a repertoire of at least 20 visually dissimilar words is achieved, selection is introduced on the basis of a named constituent letter, in particular initial or final letters. For example, the patient is presented with the four flash-cards *speak*, *along*, *pass*, *name* and instructed to point to the one that ends with *s*.

Step 5: Pairs and then groups of visually similar words are next presented; for example, *shop-stop*, *bed-bat*, *beer-bean*, *little-letter*. Note that the habit of systematic left to right search must be promoted from the beginning.

In common with all treatment programmes, the therapist is guided in the choice of materials and task complexity by the success of the patient. If, for example, the objective is to introduce longer or visually dissimilar words, then only two foils would be presented. But if the objective is to improve left to right search, then six or more words which are known to be easily identified would be presented. The principle of dropping back to an easier level of task difficulty when incorporating more complex material and, conversely, using familiar material when the task is more demanding, holds throughout all stages of treatment. A high level of success, flexibility of presentation, and continuous practice are all essential for optimum learning and to maintain the patient's confidence and motivation.

Stage II

Stage II involves: phoneme-grapheme correspondence; consonant cluster and vowel digraphs; recognition and reading aloud of orthographically regular words; print size 48 pt. to 24 pt.

Stage I will have established sufficient visual letter discrimination to allow for the introduction of phonic analysis.

Step 1: Remind the patient of the sounds which correspond to the following letters: b, c, d, f, g, h, j, k, l, m, n, p, q, (qu), r, s, t, v, w, y, z, sh, ch, th; (wh ph are introduced in Stage III) and the short vowels a, e, i, o, u. Mnemonics may be used, for example /e/ for egg. However, mastery of grapheme-phoneme correspondence is not required before proceeding to:

Step 2: Following the procedure described in Stage I, Steps 3 and 4, present flash-cards for selection by letter *sound*, not name. (Recognition of words is not essential, but is desirable). When the patient is consistently successful proceed to:

Step 3: Introduce specially prepared word lists typed on a six-pitch typewriter (extra large typeface) or printed with dry transfer lettering (24 pt.). If handwritten, the style must be uniform and clear and black fibre-tip pen should be used. Each list should illustrate a spelling rule or should vary in only one or two features. Words should be orthographically regular.[3] The patient reads each word aloud, following the therapist's model in phonologically sounding out any word which is not immediately recognized. An example list follows:

[3] Spelling rules, and lists of examples are found in: Hornsby, B. and Shear, F. (1980) Alpha to Omega: The A to Z of Teaching Reading and Spelling. London: Heinemann Educational Books.

bet	band	nine	sit
let	hand	side	sin
wet	sand	time	wit
get	land	hire	win

Step 4: Introduce consonant blends as described in Step 3

spot	best	flag	glad
spill	nest	flash	clap
spin	chest	flan	crash
spine	west	flat	tramp

Step 5: Material is devised to draw attention to the ends of words. Lists may now be ordered horizontally as well as vertically. Note that there is overlap with Stage III Step 2.

cook	cooked	cooking	cooker
shop	shopped	shopping	shopper
like	liked	liking	likes
arrive	arrived	arriving	arrives

Step 6: This involves the recognition and reading aloud of grammatically simple sentences using the split-sentence technique in a substitution-drill format. For instance, *Alan went to the bank*, is printed on a strip of card. Each word is cut out and the order jumbled. The patient first practices selecting the words named by the therapist and then reassembles the original sentence. Alternative words are then provided on cards and the procedure repeated with other combinations, for example, *Mary Fred drove ran shops town*, until reading aloud is fluent.

Step 7: Home practice can include sorting flash-cards into piles on the basis of initial or final letter and also into alphabetical order. Word recognition is not necessary for these tasks.

Stage III

This stage introduces: orthographically complex words; compound and complex sentences; phrase level scan; print size 36 pt. to 14 pt. This stage continues the development of word analysis using polysyllabic and orthographically complex words. The perception of letters in groups is facilitated by presentation of word lists which systematically vary consonants, consonant clusters and vowel combinations. This allows the patient to focus on one changing feature against a practiced and therefore increasingly familiar pattern of letters.

Step 1: Lists of single-element words demonstrating the common long vowels, vowel digraphs, and vowel-consonant digraphs are read aloud by the patient. Recourse to phonic sounding out (following a model) is usual at first, but later becomes subvocal and then redundant. Some examples follow:

been	read	boil	pain	born	park
green	team	coin	drain	short	card
queen	each	soil	wait	sport	smart
three	speak	voice	paid	torn	farm

Step 2: Affixes are used to introduce two-element words; for example, suffixes -er, -ing, -ed, -ly; prefixes un-, re-, be-, dis-. Presentation should be in columns across the page so that reading is practiced from left to right as well as from top to bottom. Examples are:

prefer	pretend	pretext	pre*ce*de
return	refer	repair	restore
dislike	dismay	disdain	disgust
behind	before	ben*ea*th	bel*ie*ve

It will now be evident that direct sounding out is inadequate for word recognition. Not only are phonemes represented by more than one spelling (see words in italics above), but often the same letter combinations may be pronounced in various ways, for example, slough, cough, rough. Although there are rules which account for many peculiarities of spelling, mastery of these is not necessary for reading. The alexic patient needs some conscious knowledge of phonics as a cue for word recognition, and to unravel errors that arise from visual misperception; but the emphasis at this stage is on training the eye to detect patterns in the letter sequences. Print may now be reduced in size; 14 pt. is recommended (size in books for the partially sighted); but patients will usually indicate the size, spacing and density which they perceive most comfortably.

Step 3: Less common letter combinations are practiced. For instance:

chemist	comb	antique	Bible
Christmas	thumb	cheque	visible
mechanic	plumber	physique	sensible
school	lamb	unique	horrible

Step 4: Compound and polysyllabic words are introduced.[4] At first examples may be written on cards and then divided into their separate elements for reassembly. For example:

foot ball	ever green	dis miss al	re port ed
footpath	waterfall	dismissive	departed
footsteps	bedroom	dismissing	imported
footloose	cardboard	dismissed	exporting

Step 5: The split sentence technique described in Stage II is used with longer and grammatically more complex sentences. The divisions should be at phrase level, not between words. The patient scans each phrase, simultaneously moving a finger or marker along the line before reading aloud. When a 'problem' word occurs, the patient should be encouraged to look at the print ahead (which may or may not be recognized), before returning to examine the constituent letters of the 'problem' word. As scanning improves, information in the periphery of vision may be used to arrive at correct identification.

---

[4] Spelling books are useful sources of polysyllabic words. The following are recommended (a) *Fowler's Scientific Spelling*, Books I–IV., MacDougall Educational Company Ltd, 30 Royal Terrace, Edinburgh; (b) *Basic Word List*, Schonell, F. J. and Schonell, F. E., Macmillan; (c) *Easy Steps in English Spelling*, Step One and Step Two, A. Wheaton and Company, Exeter.

Step 6: Dictated and spontaneous material in the patient's own handwriting is used as in Step 5.

Step 7: The large-print books for the partially sighted are used to develop reading of connected prose. Access to a Direct Image Copier (which increases or reduces the size of the reproduction) will extend the choice of material to suit the individual's tastes and interests. Some early-reader schemes provide the necessary print size as well as the repetition of vocabulary which helps improve recognition speed. Provided the patient has confidence in the clinician and the rationale of the treatment, apparently childish material will be tolerated.

The procedure is as follows. First, the selected passage is read aloud by the therapist. Next, units of phrase length are exposed for the patient to observe silently while the therapist again reads aloud. The surrounding print should be masked out with cards or a 'window' may be cut into a card. Finally, the patient reads through the complete passage at least twice, aloud. Clinical experience shows that this does not lead to rote learning or guessing behaviour, but helps the patient extend recognition span and gain confidence in visual discrimination. The patient should *not* be quizzed on the content at this stage. Some alexics show impairment of immediate visual and auditory memory. As this will affect their ability to make predictions, they should be encouraged to rehearse subvocally. As accuracy of identification improves, the chunking of groups of words and the assimilation of greater amounts of information becomes possible. Abstraction of the literal meaning is not a problem, but all patients are considerably frustrated by the restricted comprehension imposed by a slow rate of reading.

Step 8: Home practice can include copying, using the look – cover – write – check procedure. Words may be sorted into the order of entry in a dictionary. Passages may be searched, underlining, for example, all three-letter words.

Stage IV

This stage works towards: development of reading subskills; establishment of functional reading.

Up to this point the emphasis has been on the more mechanical aspects of decoding which underpin the reading process. The objective is now to establish limited but functional reading with comprehension. This requires the patient to develop a range of subskills which include speed and accuracy in recognizing words in a variety of print types and sizes; an increased recognition span; ability to look ahead and check back so that the normal sense of linguistic probabilities can operate; to follow along a line of print to the end, and then on to the next line; to use cues offered by punctuation; and finally, to retain literal meaning in memory so that higher levels of interpretation are accessible. Development of these subskills is facilitated by the following:

(i) continued use of large print;
 (At this stage of recovery print size does not necessarily alter the rate of reading. However, patients report that they feel more comfortable with large print).

(ii) orienting strategies, such as placing a coloured dot at the beginning and end of lines, and drawing a margin around the area to be studied in a newspaper;
(iii) using a card marker to expose one line of print;
(iv) moving a pen or finger *speedily* along the line;
(v) developing the patient's knowledge of compensatory strategies, so these will become self-generating, for example, checking ends of words, using phonic cues, etc.;
(vi) continued revision of work done in previous stages but with emphasis on automaticity and speed; a stopwatch can be used and records kept, so that patients can compete against themselves;
(vii) advanced search and detection exercise to improve visual scan, for example, pointing to words named at random from a line of print, tracking a spot of light from a pencil torch across a page horizontally, vertically and diagonally; simple proof-reading, etc., the patient should become conscious of the number of eye fixations made, and voluntarily try to reduce them;
(viii) listening to a text read aloud or pre-recorded, while simultaneously following the print;
(ix) using the exercises for reading comprehension commonly adopted for treatment of aphasics, for example, reading a passage and answering questions; punctuation exercises; the Cloze procedure;[5]
(x) filling in application forms and documents.

By now an increasing amount of time will be spent using the patient's own choice of material. Reading aloud will have been replaced by subvocalization, with the goal of developing beyond the stage where conscious verbal mediation is required, to the point where word groups are assimilated as thoughts.

It would be misleading to suggest that any of the patients treated by the method described have achieved anything approaching their former levels of fluency. Typically, they are reduced to a slow, deliberate rate of reading. They can no longer skim through a dictionary or telephone directory, casually read through a newspaper or magazine to pick out the gist of the story, or search through a book or catalogue to locate information for further study. Even for the well motivated and hard-working individual reading remains an arduous activity.

Treatment is usually discontinued with the mutual recognition that performance has plateaued, or that a level has been achieved which meets basic needs. Two out of five patients who were seen for follow-up about a year after regular treatment had been discontinued, had regressed to a word-by-word attack. None used eye-tracing or deciphered by oral spelling. One highly intelligent civil servant who took early retirement because of his disability, subsequently undertook a commercial speed-reading course, and was continuing to report improvement two years later. At the time he began treatment, nine months post-onset, his reading was limited to large-print letters and a few common words. Another patient is currently reading approximately 60 words per minute.

---

[5] In the Cloze procedure words are deleted from a text at regular intervals and the patient is required to fill in the gaps.

Concluding comments

The empirically based techniques described in this chapter were developed for the treatment of a distinctive type of reading disorder which is rarely encountered in clinical practice. The programme has limited application to other forms of acquired dyslexia, because its emphasis is on the manipulation of visual characteristics of the text, and the use of phonic rules as an aid to recognition. Although visual-perceptual disturbances are found in some dyslexia syndromes, manipulation of the visual distinctiveness has a negligible effect when compared to the influence of the linguistic dimensions of words on reading performance. Therefore the use of orthographically (not semantically) ordered word-lists is contra-indicated. An exception is the use of written material to remediate an impairment of phonemic hearing or a verbal dyspraxia. Attempts to re-establish reading by means of phonic analysis are unsuccessful with the majority of aphasic patients, and may even interfere with the development of more fruitful reading strategies.

The behaviour and responses of the pure alexic suggest that the disorder stems from interference with the ocular-motor and visual strategies of reading. A basic element appears to be a disturbance in the perception and discrimination of the distinctive features of graphic symbols. This is alleviated to some extent by increasing print size. There also seems to be a reduced field of effective vision; on the evidence of the literature this can be only partly explained by visual-field defects and the phenomenon of visual extinction. Improved letter discrimination brings an increase in the number of elements perceived. This can lead to fixing on a distinctive cluster of letters and consequent wrong prediction which, in connected text, produces delays and confusion rather than oral reading errors. The confusion is compounded by failure to make the normal eye recourses which in turn interferes with recognition of the succeeding words; but it rarely leads to the chain of misreadings which is characteristic of the fluent aphasic.

Some alexic patients have difficulty in grasping the theme of text, over and above the extraction of literal meaning. Other alexics show a remarkable grasp of textual sense; they display a capacity to generate expectations which should guide their processing, yet they remain 'print-bound', unable to select the most significant words and falling short of normal fluency.

Clinical experience of the treatment programme outlined here indicates a more optimistic prognosis following intervention than is suggested in the current literature. However, in view of the variety and flexibility of the word-recognition processes, and the many cues offered in printed text, the question remains why greater success is not achieved.

Pure alexia offers a unique opportunity to study a breakdown in the reading process which may be independent of the linguistic and cognitive impairments found in other acquired dyslexias. Better understanding of the nature of the deficit will help the therapist to develop and improve the rationale and methods of treatment; it will also advance knowledge of the component dynamics of normal reading.

14

Aspects of acquired dysgraphia and implications for re-education

Frances M. Hatfield

Introduction: rationale of new classification of disorders of written language

A recent development in the study of acquired disorders of written language is the use of information-processing models. These aim to identify the routes involved in the normal processes of reading or writing and to track down the point of interruption in the flow in cases of impairment following brain damage. This approach is leading to a new type of classification, with important implications for therapy.

Outline of new classification

The classification adopted here is based on the disruption or preservation of one or the other of the two principal routes or processes involved between input and output. In reading, the two main routes are (i) the grapheme-to-phoneme conversion system (which I have called here the phonological route), and (ii) the lexical-semantic route. This chapter is primarily concerned with writing, but since there are clear correspondences between reading and writing and since much more fundamental work has been carried out on reading, a brief account of the recent view of the acquired dyslexias can serve to introduce the character of this study.

Four varieties of acquired dyslexia have been described which have particular interest for cognitive psychology (Patterson 1981). In summary, these are: (i) *Phonological dyslexia*, where the phonological route is severely impaired but the lexical-semantic route well preserved; (ii) *Deep dyslexia*, where the phonological route is much more severely impaired than the lexical, but the semantic system is not intact, as evidenced by relatively frequent semantic paralexias (*table* for *chair*, *pellicle* for *atmosphere*, etc.—actual examples); (iii) *Surface dyslexia*, where it is the phonological route which is well preserved while the lexical-semantic route is impaired and (iv) *'Letter-by-letter' reading*, which is exactly what the words imply, i.e. recognition of a written word by naming the constituent letters.

To date, far less research has been devoted to acquired dysgraphia, but there have been a few important studies (e.g. Beauvois and Dérouesné 1981) which propose a model for acquired disorders of writing analogous to that described above for dyslexia. In Figure 11.1 is to be seen a much simplified version showing the two main routes involved in the normal process of reading aloud and of writing to dictation.

The following syndromes have been tentatively identified for acquired

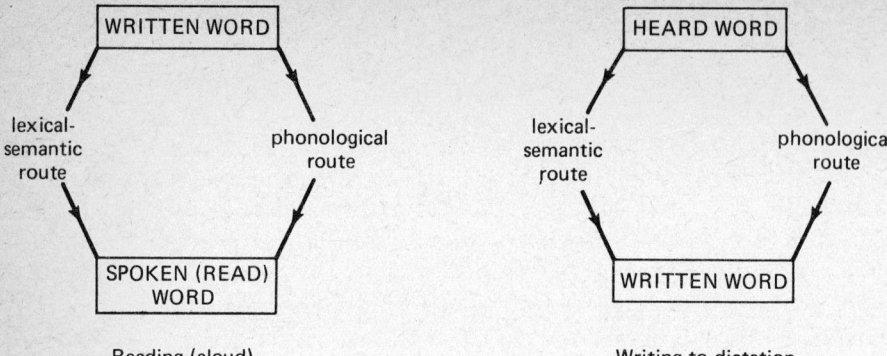

Figure 14.1 The two main routes involved in the normal processes of reading aloud and writing to dictation

dysgraphia, the characteristics of which to a certain extent mirror the forms of dyslexia mentioned above.
(i) *Phonological dysgraphia*, involving impairment of the ability to convert phonemes to graphemes but with a reasonably intact lexical system for writing; (ii) *Deep dysgraphia* (Hatfield 1980), involving impairment to both lexical-semantic and phonological processes in writing; and (iii) *Surface dysgraphia* also called *lexical* or *orthographic* agraphia (Beauvois and Dérouesné 1981; Kremin 1980; Hatfield and Patterson 1983), involving impairment of specific lexical knowledge in spelling but a reasonably intact system for translating a phonological code into a graphemic representation.

Use of new diagnostic tests for dysgraphia

This study concerns the application of tests originally developed for the analysis of dyslexia in an attempt to validate the classification of dysgraphia proposed above. It was hoped that this more sensitive classification would both lead to a better understanding of the nature of individual patients' problems and, subsequently, to the design of more effective therapy.

Description of subjects and tests

The subjects

All four subjects had been reasonably proficient at spelling before their cerebral insult. All had sustained their insult more than a year previously (range $1\frac{1}{2} - 15$ years) and were deemed beyond the stage of substantial spontaneous recovery. All were formerly right-handed.
(1) B.B., age 43, former wholesaler in greengroceries. Average education. Embolic CVA two years before the investigation. Right hemiparesis. Global aphasia with Broca-type speech and moderate impairment of verbal compre-

hension. His reading aloud, which was quite good relative to other verbal skills, was of the deep dyslexic type (Patterson 1981). Writing, both to dictation and in confrontation naming, was extremely poor, but had begun to improve just before the investigation.

(2) D.E., age 26, was assistant store-keeper in a pharmaceutical firm and able to hold down this job in spite of handicaps. Average education. Extensive left-hemisphere damage, implicating frontal and temporal lobes, following left internal carotid artery occlusion (traumatic neck injury) at age 16. Right hemiparesis. Reduced, agrammatic speech which had improved throughout the years with rather infrequent speech therapy. Comprehension good at time of testing. His reading was quintessentially deep dyslexic and has been described in detail by Patterson (1978, 1979) and Patterson and Marcel (1977). Reading much better than writing, which was poor.

(3) P.W., age 72, a former local-government officer, who suffered a cerebrovascular accident 15 years before this study. Right hemiparesis. CAT scan showed damage to frontal, temporal and parietal lobes. Broca-type speech, like D.E.'s, but with even more severe and intractable agrammatism. Reading typically deep dyslexic (see Patterson and Marcel 1977, Morton and Patterson 1980b); he had invented a number of strategies to access function words. Writing remained very poor.

(4) T.P., age 51. Formerly senior radiographer. Subarachnoid haemorrhage from angioma one and a half years before investigation affecting left temporo-occipital region. Transient hemiparesis only; permanent right homonymous hemianopia. Fluent aphasia with severe anomia and comprehension loss, which improved gradually. Unlike the first three subjects, connected writing was her first verbal modality to return; this was characterized by word-finding difficulties and spelling errors. Her reading skill improved from almost total loss to a fair performance following a period of intensive therapy: she then read mainly phonically, occasionally substituting letter-names for phonemes.

The first three subjects wrote with some facility with their left hand. B.B., occasionally, and P.W., frequently, used writing of single words spontaneously as a strategy to facilitate oral word-retrieval.

T.P. was the only one of the four to receive regular therapy for writing in the period immediately preceding the investigation. Attempts to improve spelling had been suspended some years previously for P.W. and D.E. since all the usual methods, e.g. training in phonics, had failed; little therapy had been given to B.B. for writing since he had many more urgent problems of communication. However, use of fragments of writing and drawing to aid word-retrieval and communication were at all times encouraged for these four patients.

The tests

All tests concerned writing simple words to dictation. Subjects were requested to repeat each word before trying to write it. None had any difficulty in repetition of words of one or two syllables. In the case of homophones, the words were given in a context and then again once or twice on their own. There was no time limit. The subjects indicated themselves when they wished to proceed to the next item. The first test compared writing of content words with function words, matched for length and frequency. An additional subtest compared content words of high imageability with those of low imageability (Richardson 1976b). Twenty-six items of each sort were used. Criteria for imageability were those used by Patterson and Marcel (1977) and the two sets were balanced as well as possible for length and frequency. A further test compared writing of real words and non-words, matched for length and phonemic structure. Any reasonable spelling was accepted for the non-words.

The last test of this investigation compared words deemed of 'regular' spelling with words of irregular spelling. The question of appropriateness of the terms 'regular' and 'irregular' for English spelling is a complicated one and will receive comment in the concluding section. For the test, the words selected were either perfectly regular (like *billet* and *spade*), or unambigiously irregular (like *bury, built* and *sew*). The groups of words were approximately matched for length and frequency.

Results

Responses of the four subjects were considered in their quantitative and qualitative aspects.

Quantitative results

Table 14.1 shows the results of three tests.

B.B., P.W. and D.E. show a striking superiority in writing content words over function words. T.P.'s overall performance is much better and shows a less marked effect in the same direction. Two points should be noted: the function-word list contains a higher proportion of words with irregular spelling, such as

Table 14.1: Results of tests for dysgraphia

Subject	*Correct spelling of content and function words to dictation (N=60)*		*Correct spelling of real words and non-words to dictation (N=20)*		*Correct spelling of words with regular and irregular spelling to dictation (N=22)*	
	Content	Function	Real words	Non-words	Regular	Irregular
B.B.	20	4	2	0	1	1
P.W.	20	5	4	0	6	7
D.E.	25	6	10	0	4	4
T.P.	57	48	18	18	12	9

whose, once, does and *though* than the content word list; furthermore, a number of the content words are general, and non-specific, such as *put, set, way*. There are reasons for surmising that T.P. might have achieved a higher score for function words, giving less difference between the two lists, had the two lists been more closely matched for regularity of spelling; also that the first three subjects, in particular P.W. and D.E., might have had greater success in writing content words had there been a higher proportion of more specific, concrete items, therefore showing an even greater discrepancy between the lists. For the test comparing content words of high imageability and low imageability, B.B. and P.W. achieved too few correct words of either type for significant comparison. This list was considerably more difficult *prima facie* than the Contentives *vs* Functors list and contained such words as: *knowledge, magazine* and *silhouette*. D.E. wrote eight words of high imageability correctly out of 26, but only one out of 26 of low imageability. T.P.'s scores were 17/26 and 14/26 for high imageability and low imageability, respectively. Here again, a steep gradient in performance is seen for D.E. between the two types of word; a slight difference only for T.P.

In the test comparing writing of real words and non-words, B.B. and P.W. had little success with the real words (two and four correct, respectively) and no success with non-words. In other tasks during this period, these two subjects had never been observed to succeed with non-words, whereas from time to time they wrote real words quite correctly. B.B.'s attempts at real words in the test were slightly more successful than for non-words in terms of numbers of correct letters, but it is only possible to speak of tendencies. However, D.E.'s results are more conclusive. These patients contrasted greatly with T.P., who had the same number of correct responses (18/20) for non-words as words (see Table 14.1).

In the last test, writing to dictation of words with regular and irregular spelling (see also Table 14.1), B.B. again had little success with either sort. P.W. managed six regular words correctly and seven irregularly spelt words, including *hymn, laugh* and *debt*. T.P. was slightly more successful with the regularly spelt words and it should be noted that a few months earlier, on a similar test, the difference was much more marked (78 per cent of regular words against 41 per cent irregular).

Qualitative results

The form of the errors can tell more about the way in which the subject is trying to process the information than mere statistics. The tests carried out so far show B.B., D.E. and P.W. to have characteristics of the type designated by the author and others 'deep dysgraphia' on analogy with deep dyslexia. Furthermore, analysis of their errors shows that visual, semantic and derivational errors can be found for all the three (as found by Marshall and Newcombe 1973, for deep dyslexia).

Among the errors collected from the tests so far administered are quite a number which show a visual similarity, some semantic paragraphias and 'derivational' paragraphias. Examples of responses with visual similarity include *injury → injuner, soul → sead* (B.B.); *spade → spake* (P.W.); of semantic paragraphias *stove → cooking* (P.W.), *sum → add* (D.E.); of derivational paragraphias, *whose → who* (B.B.); *built → builds* (P.W.); *called → calling* (D.E.). All three subjects made a number of responses with little visual or auditory resemblance to the stimulus, e.g. *part → people, take → nash, state → maneth*.

Among the conclusions to be drawn for all three subjects is a severe impairment of the phonological route. The disastrous results on the test of writing to dictation simple non-words, which the three patients were able to repeat without difficulty, provides strong evidence of this, particularly since the patients managed a certain number of simple real words. The importance of semantic content as a factor is shown by the superior performance on content words over function words. Moreover, not only were more of the content words correctly spelt in dictation but there were significant differences in the way they were tackled. More instances of total inability to proffer any written representation (omissions) attached to function words and the erroneous responses were more deviant (e.g. in terms of initial letter correct). For P.W. there were a couple of instances where a function word evoked a content word homophone in response: *our → hour, would → wood*.

Response to dictated non-words by B.B. and P.W. was fairly chaotic, e.g. B.B., *feps → roehse, foon → raft*; P.W., *bams → Hoo, helt → Lear*. However, P.W. sometimes tried to make a real word out of a non-word, although warned that many of the items in the task were not actual words.

There are differences between the three in the proportions of the types of errors. B.B. made proportionately more errors which could be considered visual than the other two. In some cases these involve reversals, either vertical or lateral, affecting both single letters and letter-sequences. P.W. made more semantic errors than B.B. Both these patients made some attempt at most of the test items, apart from the function words. D.E. differed in responding in an all-or-none way; typically, he wrote a response correctly and without hesitation, or else he was unable to suggest any component letter. Thus he made very few actual errors.

Both B.B. and P.W. tackled the test items slowly and deliberately, which, particularly for P.W., did not reflect a problem of penmanship. A striking characteristic was their frequent writing of a response word in an abnormal letter order. Mostly, B.B. began with the first letter or the first two letters, then left a gap and wrote what he intended to be the last letter, or the last two, leaving the middle letter or letters —which were very often vowels—to the last. P.W. generally indicates by dots the places where he thinks there should be letters. B.B. simply leaves a space of varying size. It seems likely that both for B.B. and P.W. this represents an attempt to reconstruct a visual image (much as one might do a simple jigsaw puzzle beginning with the frame and gradually filling in the central pieces), rather than a grapheme-by-phoneme representation of a phoneme sequence. The same phenomenon was reported by Hatfield and Weddell (1976) for two other cases. (See also G.F., reported by Morton 1980.) If observed by other investigators, it has seldom been reported.

In the course of the tests it was additionally noted that where the three patients, B.B., D.E. and P.W., had difficulty with certain function words they were often able to write a homophonic content word without hesitation, e.g. *him* (wrong), *hymn* (right); *our* (wrong), *hour* (right).

Other observations of the same kind were made in the course of tasks other than the above tests. For instance, B.B. failed to write the word *been* in a sentence dictation, but was able to write *bean* (the vegetable) without hesitation on the same occasion. This provides further evidence of the importance of semantic and syntactic factors in success in writing a dictated word. It furthermore testifies to a failure to use the phoneme-to-grapheme conversion system which normal people are able to operate and which there is strong evidence that the subjects were able to operate pre-morbidly. The pattern was reflected in reading behaviour. B.B. had difficulty in reading *which*, but was able to read *witch*, and this had been utilized once or twice to facilitate or 'deblock' *which*. P.W. had long utilized certain strategies of this sort in reading, for instance the name *Don* (derived from Donald Bradman, a famous cricketer of the 1930s) to access the written word *on* (Morton and Patterson 1980a and b).

The reactions of T.P. were very different. She attempted to write 100 per cent of the words: the auditory contour of the individual words was preserved, with very few exceptions. On the whole she produced a plausible representation of the stimulus word within the orthographic patterns of the English language. Her initial letters are correct with one minor exception. Her failure is in her inability to select the correct lexical form. Some of her response words are homophones (*pear → pair, seize → sees*), in spite of context given. By far the greatest number of her errors are 'homophonic' representations of the stimulus word where the response is a non-word with a plausible spelling pattern (e.g. *creed → cread, injury → ingerry, ghost → goast*). Her substituted spelling is sometimes more regular than that of the target word (e.g. *silhouette → silluet, journal → jurnal, borough → burrer*), but not always (*mode → moed, sole → sowl*). There is a small group of errors where 'letter-by-letter' writing is the best explanation: e.g. *accuracy → aquracy, treat → tret, break → brake, doe → doo*. There are a few cases of faulty application of the 'final *e* rule', e.g. *pans → panes*. There are altogether only about four instances where it is difficult to find a model or analogy in English orthography (e.g. *some → soom, mayor → meure*), of which there is only one involving a consonant (*flaw → fraw*).

The proportions of errors on the different tests and the nature of the errors identify two contrasting types of writing breakdown. The patients B.B., P.W. and D.E. share the feature of severe impairment of the phonological route in writing to dictation and of partial sparing of the lexical-semantic route. T.P., on the other hand, is still able to analyse words into their constituent phonemes and operate a simple phoneme-to-grapheme conversion system, although she lacks the lexical knowledge of which one of a number of possible graphemic representations to select when there are ambiguities (e.g. should one write *toad*, tode, towed, toed or toughed?).

The importance of the semantic dimension in successful writing for B.B., P.W. and D.E. and the lack of importance of this factor for T.P. (who can write simple non-words as well as simple words) is another major distinction.

Therapy suggested for contrasting problems in dysgraphia

The test results, combined with the error analysis, show a profound contrast between the problems of the two types of patient. Using the simple model proposed in the first section of this chapter, the principal deficits of the two types are shown in Figure 14.2 by broken lines; the routes which continue to function relatively well are also shown.

It is abundantly clear that the assets and deficits of the two 'groups' (here only one representative of surface dysgraphia is described, but there are others both in our case-load and in the literature) are fundamentally different and it follows that their therapy must differ fundamentally.

Goal of therapy for a group of three deep dysgraphics

Reactions to various tests had shown that the patients B.B., P.W. and D.E. had a specific difficulty in writing function words and certain other words low in semantic content. Among the function words were certain items—locational prepositions, verbal auxiliaries and pronouns—which are important elements in everyday communication. An immediate aim was to improve the ability to spell such words as *in, over, has, was, he, him* and *her*. The phenomenon that the patients, as a group, had been observed on occasion to write a homophonic content word, when unable to write the corresponding function word (*inn* but not *in*, *over* in cricket), but not *over*, a preposition, etc.) has been described; it has also been noted that this had been seen, both in writing and reading, to facilitate access to the target word, on occasion. With these patients, the process of phoneme-to-grapheme conversion had seriously broken down and attempts to reconstruct it directly had failed. On the positive side was their ability to write a number of concrete words to dictation. To that was added the occasionally observed ability to write the contentive, or more concrete, member of a homophonic doublet but not the functor member. This represents a definite skill which the patient has retained and therapy should take cognizance of such facts in following the principle of con-

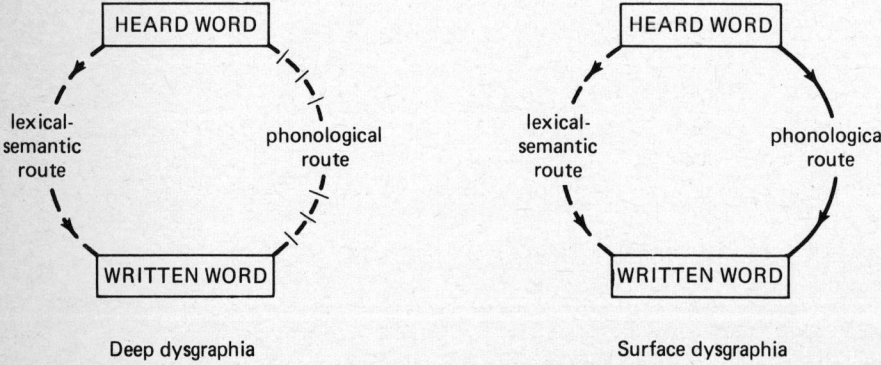

Figure 14.2 Disturbance of writing to dictation after cerebral lesion

solidating and extending the patient's residual linguistic skills (Hatfield and Elvin 1978; Hatfield 1979).

A limited number of function words were selected for practice, on the grounds of utility and of the existence of homophonic or quasi-homophonic content words to act as links in spelling: seven locational prepositions, six verbal auxiliaries and five pronouns. If the patient had no strategy of his own for retrieval of the graphic form, a link word was suggested. It was necessary for the patient to be able to write this link word without difficulty. The link words were different for individual subjects. For example, P.W. had already chosen the name *Donald* or *Don* for the preposition *on*, but the other two subjects preferred the name *Ron*. For the preposition *over*, P.W., a great cricket enthusiast, chose the cricket term *over*, but for B.B., who had no interest in cricket, the name of a village which he knew well (*Over*) was proposed. D.E. chose the word *history* to access the pronoun *his*, whereas B.B. preferred *Histon*, the name of a nearby village. All three used the word *hymn* as a strategy for the pronoun *him* and *bean* (as in *runner bean*) for *been*. There were similar strategies for all the remaining function words. The exercises described below formed but one part of each patient's total plan of language rehabilitation. This chapter is confined to quite circumscribed goals of re-education, the methods used, their outcome and their underlying rationale.

Method of working

The first stage was association of the link word with the target word. A small number of function words was chosen for practice at each session and therapist and patient worked gradually through the prepositions, the auxiliaries and the pronouns. The corresponding content word (link word), often accompanied by a little sketch, was dictated first, and next a sentence was dictated containing the target function word, which had to be written immediately under the link word. In the beginning, the prior writing of the link word did not result in correct writing of the target word in every case. After two or three sessions of this practice, with home practice in between, the next stage was reached, consisting of direct dictation of a short sentence containing the function word. The subject was allowed, and encouraged, to write the link word himself in the right-hand margin of the page if he needed this help. This stage was supplemented by homework where the subject had to fill in gaps in sentences corresponding to situations or contexts. The task here obviously extended further than retrieval of a written form to dictation to retrieval of the written word *per se*. The target words were tested periodically.

It was found necessary to give constant brief revision of earlier batches of items while simultaneously focusing more intensively on a new batch, especially for B.B.

Goal for a patient with surface dysgraphia

The therapy for T.P., a surface dysgraphic, followed completely different lines. It has been seen that she can and does operate a simple graphemic transcription phoneme by phoneme but that she has lost the more complicated rules of spelling and the memory of many spelling patterns which depend on the lexical aspect of the word. Her therapy for the period of the investigation had two aims: (i) application of the rule of doubling the consonant to preserve the quality of the vowel (*rat, ratting, sloppy,* etc.) and (ii) reacquisition of the spelling of three groups of words with the pure vowels or diphthongs /eɪ/, /i/ and /ou/ represented in different spellings—i.e. two different ways of writing the phoneme /eᵘ/ (e.g. *pain-pane*) two different spellings of /i/ (e.g. *meat-meet*) and three different spellings of /ou/, e.g. *road, rode, rowed*. For the Double Consonant rule, explanations and exercises were given for practice in the clinic and at home. For the different spelling patterns, or orthographic groups of words, a 'key-word' was given for each group, being a word which she knew fairly reliably how to write (for instance, the word *boat* as the key-word or mnemonic for the group *road, oak, soak, foam,* etc.). It was partly a question of memorizing and partly a question of finding a strategy for fixing and associating a somewhat arbitrary spelling pattern.

Outcome of therapy

It is not easy to evaluate the results of this type of 'therapeutic experiment' with severely impaired patients in simple figures without a few reservations and qualifications. One certainly would not aim at mastering the names of common objects with 100 per cent success, still less, subtleties such as the writing of function words, by patients with residual agrammatism like B.B., P.W. and D.E. Improvement, rather than mastery, would be a more realistic aim. The observation that the use of certain content words frequently helped the deep dysgraphic patients to write function words led to the initiation of systematic exercises to reinforce this strategy and afterwards it could be seen that the patients had some success in writing the function word directly. By 'directly' is to be understood, without having the linking content word dictated to them first; certainly, the three patients continued to use these strategies themselves 'in their heads'; sometimes they would hesitate for a longish time over a function word and when asked how they had finally managed to write that word they would explain that it was by dint of one of the rehearsed strategies (for example, thinking of the in(n)—which they often called 'pub'—in order to arrive at the spelling of the preposition *in*).

Table 14.2 gives some results for B.B., whose therapy was in many ways the most straightforward and certainly the most regular and intensive, although his practice with the therapist was limited to twice a week. Performance has been assessed at three stages: the first just before and at the moment of beginning the experiment; the second, after a couple of sessions of practice in writing the target word (function word) in a short sentence *after* writing the link word dictated by the therapist; the third stage, writing the target word 'directly' to dictation, as explained. The tests of performance were carried out on two or three sessions, so that the results represent an average performance.

B.B. encountered some difficulty of a cognitive-linguistic nature in dealing with pronouns. A larger number of items were introduced at the beginning but some of these had to be eliminated on the grounds of conceptual difficulty or lack of a suitable link word. Similarly with prepositions and auxiliaries, a few of the original

Table 14.2: Writing of function words to dictation: improvement in course of re-education

Patient B.B.	7 prepositions	Correct responses 6 auxiliaries	5 pronouns	Total	
1st stage	7/21	6/17	4/13	17/51	34%
2nd stage	13/17	10/20	8/11	31/40	61%
3rd stage	15/21	16/20	9/12	40/63	63.5%

Patient D.E.	Correct responses Total (7 prepositions, 6 auxiliaries, 5 pronouns)
1st stage	49%
2nd stage	68%
3rd stage	67%

batch had to be abandoned. These eliminated items are *not* included in the scores.

It must be realized that Stage 2, when the therapist provides the strategy or reminds the patient of it, is inherently easier than Stage 3, when he has to remember the strategy himself or else directly access the function word.

D.E. was not able to attend as regularly as B.B. In general, he was quicker to learn new skills and strategies in spite of his long-standing handicaps. His therapy followed approximately the same course as B.B.'s. His data are fewer, so the figures for the three groups of function words have been amalgamated (see Table 14.2).

D.E. was able to use the type of strategies indicated above to access the written form of the prepositions after quite a brief explanation and demonstration. He took much longer to be able to apply the same kinds of strategy for verbal auxiliaries and pronouns.

The results of P.W.'s therapy are even more difficult to quantify, since there were some minor differences in the therapeutic method. Moreover he had used a few of the strategies described (for example *Don* or *Donald* for *on*) for a considerable time before the actual period of the experiment, in reading, occasionally in writing, and even sometimes in speech in the course of clinical tasks. In writing he would often use the whole word *Donald* and then separate the required portion by means of brackets. With prepositions which he had *not* practised before the experimental period, and for which he had not evolved strategies, he made considerable progress. After five or six sessions of systematic practice he was writing all the seven prepositions correctly nine times out of ten, almost always by means of the practised strategies.

That the progress recorded for all three subjects was not due to simple repetition of the items was indicated by frequent demonstrations of the use of a specific 'strategy' by all the three, either overtly or covertly (in the latter case they would report the use of the strategy when questioned as to how they had achieved a certain correct response).

For T.P. the goals and method of assessment were different. The procedure was more conventionally didactic and in some respects resembled common methods of teaching spelling rules and patterns to pupils of eight to ten years of age (obviously giving her words and explanations suitable for an intelligent adult). Her re-education, like that of the other three patients, is far from being completed, but progress can already be registered. This period of her therapy is divided into two stages, stage one at the beginning of systematic re-teaching of the consonant-doubling rule and of the three groups of words described above (the two tasks were not introduced at the same moment) and stage two after four or five sessions with homework in between. Her progress is indicated in Table 14.3.

Table 14.3: Results of T.P.'s therapy and practice

	Correct responses	
	Doubling of Consonant Rule	Spelling of words with phonemes /ou/, /e./, /i/
1st stage	12/20	11/20
2nd stage	16/20	17/20

Summary and concluding remarks

(1) The thrust of this chapter has been to illustrate how the findings of neuropsychological research and recent theoretical conceptions and models may be directly applied to re-education of the brain-damaged. Such data and hypotheses in the case of acquired dyslexia, in particular the type designated 'deep dyslexia', had already been put to use in therapy in our clinic: our attention had been drawn by our collaborators to the importance of the factor of concreteness and we realized that our former concentration on shortness of the word and regularity of spelling (i.e. confining the initial texts to regularly spelt three and four-letter words), and even word frequency, with 'progress' to longer, more complexly structured words, did not constitute a logical or appropriate method for deep dylexics. Instead texts which were on the whole grammatical but avoided abstract words and particles as far as possible were used to begin with. The same is now being done for secondary dysgraphia, using somewhat simplified versions of the models proposed by Morton (1980), Beauvois and Dérouesné (1981) and others. We consider this to be a happy outcome of the conflict between research and therapy.

(2) The tests used, although in need of certain modifications, served to point up profound differences between two groups of patient with acquired dysgraphia, who have often been lumped together in the past and treated by identical methods.

(3) Using a new type of classification and a new orientation it has been possible to elaborate a therapy which rests squarely on a well thought out theory and proved adapted to the problems of individual patients.

(4) The methods of remediation used had a satisfactory outcome with subjects suffering from very severe aphasia and dysgraphia.

(5) The value of so much attention to writing, especially of function words, for patients with such severe all-round verbal handicaps, might be questioned. In a brief justification it should be pointed out, firstly, that writing can consolidate and

assist oral language and, secondly, that there are some cases (Kotten 1979; Hatfield 1980) where the graphic modality is better preserved than the oral for certain function words.

(6) It might also be wondered whether the patients, in particular B.B., P.W. and D.E., with their agrammatism and comprehension problems, were able to appreciate the meaning of what they were being asked to write, or whether, on the contrary, their failure to understand certain function words were not the root of the difficulty. In fact, it was carefully controlled at each step that they did understand the target word. Moreover the therapy actually helped, indirectly, to improve both comprehension and oral expression of the grammatical classes concerned.

(7) The fourth patient, T.P., had problems of a different order from the other three, problems which are intimately concerned with analysis of a spoken word and the conversion of its constituents into a somewhat arbitrary written code. This whole problem is the subject of another paper (Hatfield and Patterson 1983). It must be remembered that the notion of 'phoneme-to-grapheme conversion rules', as described by Weigl (1972) and Weigl and Fradis (1977), applied primarily to the German language, where the spelling system is fairly regular; something much subtler is required for the intricacies of English spelling, where the writer is presented with a great number of graphic patterns of varying frequency, representing the same phoneme. This is not to say that there are not 'rules' for segments larger than single letters, 'rules' connected with morphology and 'rules' dependent on etymology, the latter probably playing a minor, if not negligible, role. For T.P. and patients like her it cannot be said that they have preserved the normal phonological route, but they have preserved some kind of phonological route which represents the patterns of English orthographic convention.

Acknowledgments
The author is indebted to the following Consultants of Addenbrooke's Hospital for permission to publish certain data on their patients: Dr O.M. Edwards (for patient B.B.), Mr J.R.W. Gleave (for patient D.E.), Dr I.M.S. Wilkinson (for patient P.W.) and Mr A. Holmes (for patient T.P.). She would like to express her appreciation to Dr J. Morton and Dr K. Patterson for helpful suggestions during the period of testing and for frank criticism of the interpretation of results, which remains, however, essentially her own. She would also like to express her gratitude to the four subjects for their willing cooperation in a 'therapeutic experiment'. The study was partly funded by the East Anglian Regional Health Authority, to which the author also acknowledges sincere thanks.

Alternative Communication Methods

The possibilities and limitations of artificial languages and communication aids in aphasia therapy are discussed in this section. Rowley presents a brief introduction to the literature on the use of artificial languages with aphasic patients and examines some of the communication aids which may be of use. Bailey describes the experimental use of an artificial language, Blissymbolics, and Enderby and Hamilton report on a trial of 'Splink', an electronic aid which has been developed for the communicatively impaired.

15

Artificial languages and communication aids in aphasia therapy

David T. Rowley

Introduction

One of the most interesting approaches to therapy for aphasic patients during the last decade involves attempting to teach them an artificial language system. This is interesting not only because, as Castro-Caldas (1975) concludes, it has shown some signs of success, but also because its theoretical basis is that cognitive abilities remain which will enable the patient to learn a language. Basso, De Renzi, Faglioni, Scotti and Spinnler (1973) have shown that even in severe aphasia certain cognitive abilities may remain virtually intact and hence potentially available to the therapist.

This possibility has been acknowledged in several other forms of therapy. Thus the ability of many aphasic patients to perceive and produce rhythmical and intonational patterns has been utilized in melodic intonation therapy (Albert, Sparks and Helm 1973). Similarly, pantomime therapy (Schlanger and Freimann 1979) makes use of the individual's ability to perceive and perform patterned movements in space, as documented by Kimura (1973) and Nebes (1973) who suggest that the non-dominant hemisphere is more specialized for this role. However, the conclusion by Goodglass and Kaplan (1963) that aphasics have a gestural deficiency, and the later work by Kimura and Archibald (1974) which shows more specifically that patients with left-hemisphere damage perform less well on imitating visually presented meaningless hand movements, indicates that the situation is more complex than outlined by Schlanger and Freimann (1979). This should obviously not be taken to imply that for some patients pantomime therapy is not a possible form of treatment. Having briefly mentioned some other forms of therapy and how they may make use of residual cognitive abilities several artificial language systems that have been used with aphasic patients will now be discussed to illustrate how they make use of these remaining abilities.

Artificial language systems

One of the earliest examples was by Glass, Gazzaniga and Premack (1973) who attempted to teach seven patients a modified version of the artificial language system originally developed by Premack (1971) for chimpanzees. This system comprises symbols cut from paper, which vary in colour, size and shape, and are functionally equivalent to words. They can be arranged to form sentences, and have the advantage that their permanency removes any problem which may arise due to the patient perhaps possessing a memory disability and thereby experiencing difficulties in dealing with transitory symbols. The individuals taught this system were able to acquire it with varying degrees of success, two progressing well enough to express and comprehend simple declarative sentences. It is interesting to note that in the initial perceptual-cognitive assessment used by the investigators very few difficulties were experienced by the patients, which may indicate that in the learning of the artificial language system there is a substrate of residual cognitive abilities which they can make use of. As Gardner, Zurif, Berry and Baker (1976) state however, this work was not primarily intended for the purpose of establishing a framework for functional communication but rather to determine to what extent basic logical capacities were spared.

In contrast the work of Gardner et al. (1976), Davis and Gardner (1976) and Baker, Berry, Gardner, Zurif, Davis and Veroff (1975) aims to do just this, that is to produce an artificial language system which can be used for communication by aphasic patients. They call this system VIC, which is an acronym for Visual Communication. The VIC system consists of index cards, three inches by five inches in size, on each of which is drawn a simple arbitrary (geometric) or representational (ideographic) form which denotes a meaningful unit. Symbols denoting conjunctions and prepositions are drawn on smaller, half-sized index cards. There are two levels on which communication can take place, which are shown in Table 15.1.

In Level 1 the patient learns three communicative functions in the following order: carrying out commands, answering questions and describing events. In Level 2 the patient receives training in the use of VIC as a means of expressing his feelings, needs and desires. These symbols are arranged in a linear left-to-right sequence to form sentences. Typically the agent of the action is at the beginning of the sentence, followed by the verb, with the objects, locations, and beneficiaries of the action appearing next. Metalinguistic markers appear before the symbol denoting the agent of action.

Of the 15 patients who were taught VIC only eight were considered to have had sufficient opportunity to master the system, the remaining seven dropping out for various reasons. Five of these eight patients reached a standard in VIC which far surpassed their performance on matching tasks in English.

A rather more informal study has been carried out by Cameron (1976). This system involved teaching an aphasic patient, who was unable to communicate verbally in any way, a number of representational symbols, viz. seven verbs and 14 nouns. The patient was taught their meanings using photographs of the objects depicted by the symbols, and appeared to learn them with very little difficulty. The next stage involved the introduction of 20 more symbols for the patient to learn. Initially this seemed to cause some confusion, and unfortunately the patient's deteriorating health ended the training.

However, Cameron found this trial successful enough to put forward a revised programme which included some arbitrary symbols which he envisaged would be taught using photographs and cartoons. Of particular interest is his proposal for establishing a means whereby a patient might move in stages from an

Table 15.1: Types of symbol used in VIC (From Gardner *et al*. 1976, 279)

Symbol type	Description	English example
Level 1		
Proper nouns (personal pronouns)	Arbitrary symbols which may double as personal pronouns	Lynn
Common nouns	Representational symbols	Glass
Verbs	Arbitrary symbols	Pick up
Prepositions	Partially representational symbols on half-sized cards	In
Conjunctions	Arbitrary symbols on half-sized cards	And
Request forms for specific information	Arbitrary symbols	Who.
Message category markers	Arbitrary symbols	?
Metalinguistic marker	Arbitrary symbol	Describe this action
Level 2		
Interjections	Arbitrary symbols on half-sized cards	True
Adjectives	Representational drawings of facial expressions, used principally with the verb 'feel'	Happy
Location and activity particles	Pictorial scenes. Used with 'when' interrogative or in simple declarative	Go home

understanding of a pictographic representation to an understanding of a corresponding arbitrary symbol, as shown in Figure 15.1.

Implications

The preceding brief account of artificial language systems raises some interesting points. Perhaps the most striking is that despite the fact that the patients tested had either no or very little communicative ability the majority were able to learn an artificial language system to some extent. The question is to what extent could they be considered to be communicating with it?

Davis and Gardner (1976) show that they are well aware of this problem and wonder whether patients view VIC as an elaborate game, as a system with general communicative potential, or as some sort of mixture of the two. It seems that the majority of patients in their study regarded VIC as a mixture of the two. Thus they used the card to request cigarettes and matches to enable them to smoke, but did not seem to be aware that VIC is potentially a communication system which can be used outside the therapeutic session. Cameron's (1976) patient does seem to have been much more aware of the communicative potential of the system he was using, as instanced by his suggesting the use of a symbol for cigarettes and matches. This may have been due to the different systems and teaching methods used, to

174 ALTERNATIVE COMMUNICATION METHODS

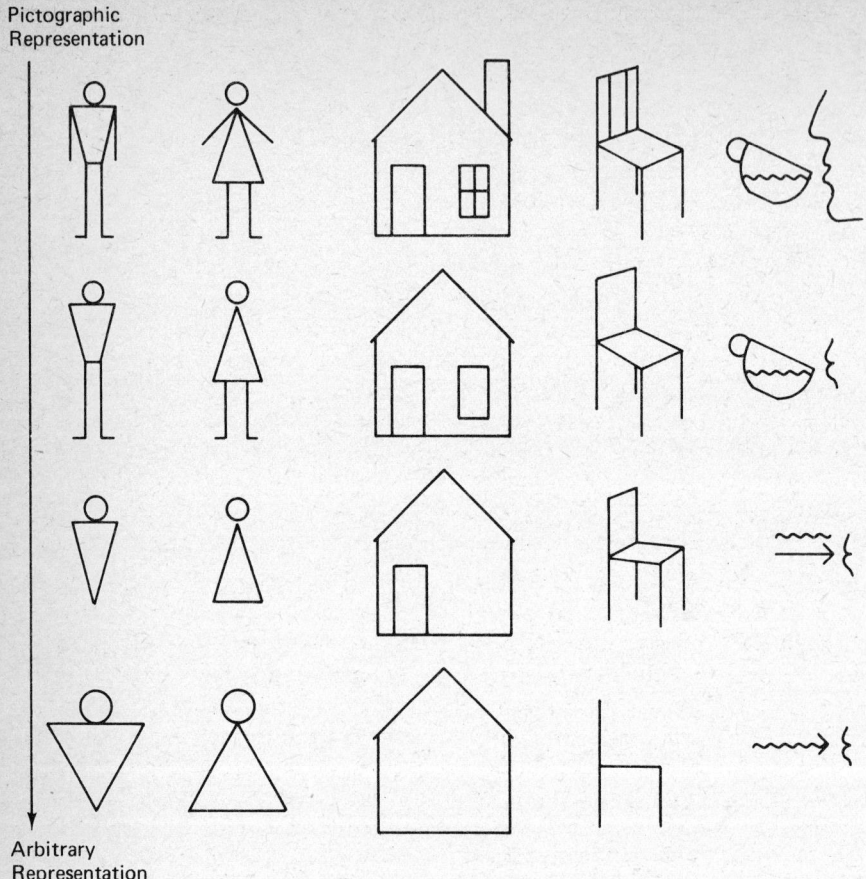

Figure 15.1 The change from a pictographic to a more arbitrary form of representation

individual differences in the patients, or to a combination of these factors. Whatever the reasons this last finding does seem encouraging. Glass *et al.* (1973) do not really address themselves to this problem, but they do believe that their observations suggest that the patients still retain the ability to learn an artificial language, which implies that it may be possible to use the system in a communicative capacity outside the therapeutic session.

The most reasonable conclusion is that many aphasic patients with severe language problems seem able to learn an artificial language system, and on certain occasions some do seem to be aware of its general communicative potential.

Closely related to this is the extent to which cognitive functioning remains unimpaired. This was the question which Glass *et al.* (1973) were particularly concerned with. The assessments they carried out, and the ability of their patients to master at least partially the artificial language system, does lead to the conclusion that certain cognitive abilities do remain. Particularly of interest here is the extent to which cognitive abilities essential to language processing may persist, even in the event of severe damage in the dominant hemisphere. There is also considerable debate concerning the location of these cognitive abilities, with an increasing amount of evidence (Czopf 1979; Pettit and Noll 1979; and Code, chapter 4 this volume) supporting the dominance-shift hypothesis, which holds that for aphasic patients the previously non-dominant hemisphere becomes increasingly important in any recovery of language abilities which may take place.

Glass et al. (1973) consider it possible that the basic cognitive mechanisms which underlie language are shared by both hemispheres, which would be consistent with the above hypothesis, since as the underlying cognitive mechanisms actually become used for learning language one might expect dominance to shift to that hemisphere where the cognitive mechanisms remain intact. If this is the case however, it may be that the finding of Gardner et al. (1976), that there is a negative correlation between patient's natural language ability and their ability to use VIC, is due to some form of interference between any residual language and the artificial language system they are attempting to learn, or it may simply reflect a general unwillingness to adopt non-standard forms of communication (see Bailey, chapter 16, this volume).

Gardner et al.'s finding is not what might be expected if the possibility is considered that learning an artificial language system may enhance the return of natural language. Unfortunately none of the studies directly consider this possibility. As the majority of the patients had received speech therapy for six months with very little improvement, and in addition had received severe damage to the dominant hemisphere, perhaps the lack of information on this possibility is not so surprising. However, the therapist may hope that if the patient is able to learn an artificial language system then this could be at least an indication that some understanding and use of natural language may return to the patients.

It may be that this hope is misplaced and that patients are able to learn an artificial language system like VIC, even to the point of regarding it as a communication system equal to natural language, but yet this ability shows no sign of returning. In this situation patients' requirements are for some artificial language system which will fulfil, at least partially, their communicative needs outside the therapy session. So far it remains to be seen if the above-mentioned artificial language systems can do this, although there are a number of technical aids which, it could be argued, partially fulfil a similar function. These aids will be discussed in the next section.

Technical aids in aphasia therapy and rehabilitation

There are a number of technical aids which may be of use to aphasia therapists and their aphasic patients. These include tape recorders, the Bell and Howell Language Master, the Canon Communicator, the Lightwriter, the Speak and Spell, the Possum Communicator, SPLINK, and various personal computers.

Obviously the use of any particular aid is only possible when it matches the needs of the patient. The tape recorder is a very versatile piece of equipment which clinicians are very familiar with, and many have discovered ways of using it in treating their aphasic patients. The Bell and Howell Language Master is a device which plays specially prepared cards which bear visual information (words and illustrations) and a two-track magnetic tape, one track usually being used by the therapist, the other by the patient. This can be used by some aphasic patients to improve their visual and auditory retention.

The Canon Communicator and the Lightwriter are very similar. Both are designed for persons who are unable to speak, and consist of a keyboard on which words can be spelled out, which then appear in written form. On the Canon Communicator they are printed on paper tape, and the device can be worn on the wrist, whereas for the Lightwriter the words appear on a display screen, and the device is less portable. Closely related to these aids is the Speak and Spell. This also consists of a keyboard on which words can be spelled, but here the output of the machine is speech. It is also easily portable. These three items of equipment may be of use for aphasic patients who have retained word-finding and spelling ability, but for one reason or another are unable adequately to produce spoken language.

The Possum Communicator is rather different. It comprises a panel of 100 cells in a 10 by 10 matrix, in each of which is a word. The user moves a light across the panel, stopping when the required word is illumined. The words in the panel can be changed by fitting a different overlay sheet, and by completing blank sheets it is possible to tailor the vocabulary for individual patients. The device is portable, but probably needs to be set down before use in many cases. It can be used by aphasic patients who retain their word-recognition ability, and if the therapist were to draw words in each cell could be used by a wider group of patients.

SPLINK (Enderby and Hamilton, chapter 17, this volume) is in some ways a similar kind of device to the above. SPLINK (an acronym for speech link) consists of an electronic keyboard on which in individual cells are 950 basic words, letters, numerals, prefixes, suffixes and elementary phrases, a total of 1024 in all. The user selects one of these by pressing the required cell. This information is then beamed by an infra-red ray to a microprocessor which is plugged into the aerial socket of a television, and appears on the screen. About 120 words can be present on the screen at any one time. It is of most use to aphasic patients who retain their word recognition ability, although it may be possible to incorporate into the display some pictures, which could increase the number of aphasic patients who would benefit from it. Although SPLINK's infra-red link to the television does increase its portability, it is not really usable without its microprocessor and a television.

The above aids are all rather specific, at least compared to personal computers. A portable computer, of which a number are now available, will certainly have advantages over the Canon Communicator and the Lightwriter, and over the Speak and Spell too, particularly if it were to possess spoken output. It would certainly have advantages as regards portability, combining keyboard and visual display in a box approximately 30 centimetres long, 15 centimetres wide and 10 centimetres deep. If each key were to have a dual function about 80 different letters and words could be used, although it is quite possible to make modifications to enable each key to have more than two functions, in which case it is starting to overlap in function with the Possum Communicator and the SPLINK. Furthermore, the personal computer has two more advantages: it is considerably cheaper because of the number produced, and it is more versatile. In addition to being used as an aid to communication for certain aphasic patients their families can make use of it as an ordinary computer, as indeed can the patient. Personal computers seem to offer a lot of potential as an aid in speech therapy for aphasic patients.

It is also worth briefly considering the form an artificial language system should take, and how it could be taught to the patient. It may be that a system like BLISS would be a possibility (see Bailey, chapter 16, this volume), although Cameron's (1976) idea that the patient may find it easier to learn arbitrary symbols if their derivation is made clear seems worth bearing in mind. The advantage of a computer now becomes even clearer, as given a suitable program it could be used not only as a communication device, but also as an aid in the initial teaching of the communication system.

Using artificial language systems in real-life situations: a conclusion

It may well be argued that artificial language systems involving communication using index cards with symbols drawn on them are of limited use outside the clinic. For the aphasic patient with a supportive family, partial or total mastery of an artificial language system would allow limited but important communication with those in the immediate environment. However, for the hospitalized patient the benefits may well be much less. Similarly this kind of system is not likely to be of much practical use outside the home.

The use of such a system in real-life situations depends on its ease of use and understanding by people who are very unfamiliar with it. As intimated in the last section, a portable computer offers one solution to this problem. If each of 40 keys on the keyboard had only a dual function this would give 80 symbols which could be used for VIC, or a similar system. The aphasic patient could then select a sequence of these keys to produce simple phrases. This is much simpler than attempting to find index cards and place them in order, and also has the advantage that the display can be more easily shown to people. Furthermore, if spoken output is produced the application of artificial language systems in real-life is even greater.

16
Blissymbolics and aphasia therapy: a case study
Stella Bailey

Introduction

Blissymbolics is one method of communication which has recently attracted attention as a possible alternative to 'natural' language in a variety of communication disorders. It is a visuographic system of logically based symbols which makes communication possible without use of the spoken or written word; although the written word does always appear with the symbol, thus making communication possible with the non-symbol user. Symbols are related to meaning either pictorially, ideographically or arbitrarily. The structure of the system enables the user to expand a small number of basic symbols into a symbol vocabulary of infinite size. Bliss has a syntax of its own which is not bound by, or to, the rules of any other language, but is also logically based (Bliss 1965).

Before any alternative is formally introduced there must be careful evaluation of the individual's abilities, needs and motivation. The family should also be considered and consulted. If they are unable to accept and encourage the aphasic's use of an alternative form of communication the success of any programme is likely to be limited.

Method

Subject

B.L. is a 55-year-old right-handed male, a scientist by profession, who suffered a CVA in January 1976 which left him with a complete right hemiplegia, severe dysphasia and an articulatory dyspraxia. A computerized tomography scan in September 1980, four years eight months post-onset, showed a large area of infarction in the left hemisphere stretching from the left mid-temporal region adjacent to the insula up alongside the left lateral ventrical almost to the vertex where there was some calcification in the superior part of the lesion. The investigation was undertaken to clarify the exact nature and extent of the lesion, no investigation having been made initially. Since onset B.L. has had no further incidents and although a pattern of regular three-weekly fits developed approximately 18 months post-onset (MPO), these were immediately and completely controlled with drugs.

Initially B.L. was unable to match the written or spoken word to an object and had only unintelligible vocalization. He had regular speech therapy from 1 MPO and daily from 2 MPO for six months. By September 1976 he could comprehend simple spoken sentences intermittently, match some words to pictures, copy words and write his own and a few object names spontaneously. The only speech was a recurrent utterance 'kiss, kiss, kiss'.

Emotionally B.L. exhibited extreme frustration and despair. He was totally aware of his failure to communicate. This, with the observation of his participation in draughts, card games and other non-verbal activities, led to the decision to make a more careful evaluation of his residual skills and difficulties with a view to introducing some alternative communication medium.

Assessment

Only 29 of the 47 sub-tests of the Minnesota Test for the Differential Diagnosis of Aphasia (MTDDA) (Schuell 1964) were attempted and he had an error score of 100 per cent on four of those, yielding a severity rating of 395 (maximum 573). The severity rating is the total error score on sections A–D (Powell, Clark and Bailey 1979). (See Table 16.1).

By contrast, his non-verbal performance was better than that of many dysphasic patients, and unique for one with his severity of language handicap. On Raven's Coloured Progressive Matrices (RCPM) he scored 100 per cent (Raven 1938a). The standard (RSPM) version was therefore administered (Raven 1938b) and he obtained a score of 55 out of a possible 60 placing him in the 95th percentile compared with a normal 56 year old male. On Koh's Block Design Test he scored 75 per cent (See Table 16.1). These results confirmed the subjective impression that an alternative to natural language therapy should be tried. Gesture or sign language were ruled out because of the hemiplegia and his demonstrably poor ability for gesture, which was both inappropriate and perseverative. Progress in written language was too slow for his apparent needs. It seemed that a system which might utilize the apparently good right hemisphere was needed.

Symbol discrimination requires good visuo-perceptual skills. The user must be able to differentiate between shapes, sizes, different orientations of the same shape and many computations of these differences. Sample symbols were introduced to test B.L.'s ability to differentiate, identify and learn to attach meaning to both pictographic and ideographic symbols. For example the symbol for house or home is the outline of a house—pictographic, the heart shape is used in any symbols to do with feelings, thus a heart alone is 'feeling' and a heart accompanied by an upward pointing arrow means 'happy'—ideographic. The results were encouraging, B.L. quickly learned about a dozen symbols.

The next step was careful preparation of B.L. and his wife. The experimental nature of the use of Blissymbolics with aphasic adults was explained and the system described and demonstrated. The need for Mrs B.L.'s support and participation in the programme was stressed.

Results

September 1976 – March 1977

The Bliss programme began in October 1976, 9 MPO, immediately following the first formal assessment (Table 16.1). Progress was measured at six-monthly intervals thereafter on the same battery of tests. B.L. attended the unit for three whole days per week for both individual and group treatment.

The aim initially was to build a symbol vocabulary of the, then standard, 100-word chart following the Blissymbolics Communication Institute programme guidelines. Some vocabulary substitutions were made more appropriate to B.L.'s needs. In the six months he learned to use the special symbol for 'opposite' to increase the available adjectives; so that, for instance, 'opposite hot' means 'cold'. He also learnt to use the action symbol to create verbs—e.g. 'action with legs' becomes 'to walk' or 'to go'—he also used the plural symbol. It took the full six months to introduce all the symbols. At this stage he used symbols in structured situations only; pictures, object and direct questions were used to stimulate output. Although encouraged from the start to point to the chart he preferred to write down the symbols.

6 to 12 months

The first reassessment was encouraging, notably the 24 per cent improvement in auditory abilities. (Table 16.1). It is however questionable whether this was the result of symbols *per se* or, the structure of the programme which dictated consistent and prolonged repetition of a limited vocabulary.

It had become apparent that a programme used to stimulate language development in children was not entirely appropriate for encouraging the recovery of language in an adult. Some of the demands made by the programme were beyond any which would normally have been thought helpful or appropriate in therapy at this stage, for instance the inclusion of so many different syntactic categories. The content of the chart was therefore modified to give a principally noun vocabulary, with symbols for 'action', 'opposite' and 'plural' being retained with interrogatives 'what', 'where', 'when' and 'how many' and pronouns 'I' and 'you', all of which B.L. understood and used in structured situations. There was evidence that he was able to generalize what he had learned. An aspect of symbols that B.L. found hardest to accept was the simplification whereby the same symbol can be interpreted differently depending on the context.

In this second stage of the programme the idea of combining symbols to create new meanings was introduced. This would have been simplified if it had not been felt necessary to adhere to Bliss which suggests that a non-standard symbol be marked by an indicator at the start and finish, and that symbols containing more than one element must express the main concept first. For example, a 'garden chair' becomes a 'chair garden' in symbols.

The emphasis at this stage was concentrated more on the encouragement of symbol output and therefore group symbol activities were introduced. The

Table 16.1: Pre-treatment and ongoing assessment on MTDDA, RSPM, and Block Design

	Sept. 76		March 77		Sept. 77		March 78		Sept. 78		March 79	
	error score	% score	error score	% score	error score	% score	error score	% score	error score	% score	error score	% score
MTDDA												
Severity Rating	395	68	339	59	339	59	312	54	297	51	287	50
Aud. comp.	75	64	47	40	68	58	50	43	36	30	40	34
Reading	76	48	69	43	69	43	61	38	59	37	61	38
Sp/Lang.	171	94	169	93	151	83	149	81	153	84	131	71
Writing	—	—	52	46	51	45	52	46	49	43	45	39
Number	11	30	6	18	14	42	7	21	6	18	5	15
RSPM												
Total	50		54		50		50		50		52	
Grade	G1+		G1+		G1+		G1+		G1+		G1+	
Percentile	95th		95th		95th		95th		95th		95th	
Block Design												
Total	100		114		126		123		130		126	
Percentage	75		85		94		92		97		94	

activities were planned for different levels of ability so that B.L. was able to work with all his fellow dysphasics and to familiarize the whole group with symbols. These activities were aimed at specific areas of treatment rather than aiming to teach the system itself. At the simplest level this might be a visual matching task. At a slightly higher level symbols assisted in the comprehension of prepositions of place, for example helping to clarify the easily confusable in/on, beside/between differences.

12 to 18 months

Despite a break in treatment of one month during the summer, when the programme was recommenced in September B.L. appeared to have retained his symbol vocabulary. On reassessment however at the end of September there was a marked reduction in his auditory comprehension score—plus 18 per cent errors—(Table 16.1) on MTDDA compared with the previous test. This decrement may have been a reflection of the emphasis placed on the expressive use of symbols in the previous six months or the possible effect of the recently developed fits, or of the drugs introduced to control them.

Two problems which had emerged during the programme were focused on during this period. B.L. frequently confused symbols which were visually dissimilar but whose written meanings were visually similar, e.g. head/hand. This suggested that he may have been trying to rely more on the written word than the symbol. A second working chart was therefore introduced without words; this made little difference to his performance.

The second problem was a sequencing and memory difficulty which made it necessary for him to try to keep a finger on each symbol in a response until it was complete. Despite the difficulties it was felt that B.L. was ready for, and needed, a larger vocabulary and planning for a 200-word chart began.

18 to 24 months

Test results in March, 1978 showed further progress; auditory comprehension had improved (Table 16.1), though not quite to the level of the previous March. More significantly however B.L. had now begun to use symbols spontaneously both at home and in treatment sessions. B.L. now began to use symbols more creatively using strategies, and 'combine' in situations he had not been taught. For example, he used the opposite symbol to change 'play' into 'work', and the action symbol freely to increase his verb vocabulary. These developments confirmed the impression that he needed a larger vocabulary of basic symbols. Again no symbol was included on the chart until he had demonstrated a full understanding and an ability to use it in a variety of structured situations.

24 to 30 months

By September, 1978 B.L. was using the complete 200 chart. He had difficulty remembering the location of some of the less frequently used symbols but given sufficient time he was generally able to complete his statements adequately. Assessment demonstrated a further improvement (plus 13 per cent) in auditory comprehension (Table 16.1)—the 3 per cent drop in the expressive language score was probably insignificant.

During this next six months B.L. changed from writing the word below the symbol, as they appeared on the standard BCI displays, to putting it above, which suggested the growing primacy of the written word as a means of communication. Further evidence for this was the mixture of words and symbols he now used for spontaneous communication. When recording his symbol output, either in speech or writing, they had always been expanded to include all function words although telegraphic sentences were the aim for B.L. At this stage he began to leave gaps in his written symbol output and where a function word might be used, he frequently wrote in 'and', 'the' or 'with', not always appropriately. Sequencing difficulties were almost exclusively at the sentence level. At the phrase level he was generally accurate.

Because of his increasing skill and confidence there were more things B.L. wished to 'say' and it was evident that if progress and motivation were to be sustained he needed a further increase in vocabulary. It was decided to try and plan for a 'definitive' chart which could accommodate a growing vocabulary without increasing the overall dimensions of the chart and avoid the rearrangement of contents.

30 months

Reassessment in March, 1979 showed a small overall improvement despite the slight increase in auditory comprehension errors (Table 16.1). This was however a 24 per cent improvement on the initial pre-Bliss performance and at a time (39 MPO) when progress would be expected to be limited.

New strategies and Bliss techniques were introduced to see whether B.L. was able to use them and a temporary layout was produced. Initially this chart contained only familiar symbols to allow him time to adjust to the reduction in symbol size and the amended layout. New symbols were added as and when he was able to understand and use them; as well as making learning easier, this allowed greater flexibility.

In June, 1979, when the main body of the new chart was almost complete, B.L. began to indicate that he no longer wished to have symbols on the chart. He had begun to rely more on the written word for his spontaneous communication and, although spelling and syntax presented a problem, he could generally convey his meaning. It was therefore agreed, after discussion with B.L. and his wife, that we adapt the chart to a word-board retaining a few of the Bliss techniques to allow for a more extensive vocabulary. Work on the Bliss programme ceased at this stage.

Discussion

Figure 16.1 illustrates the change in MTDDA scores during the programme. This

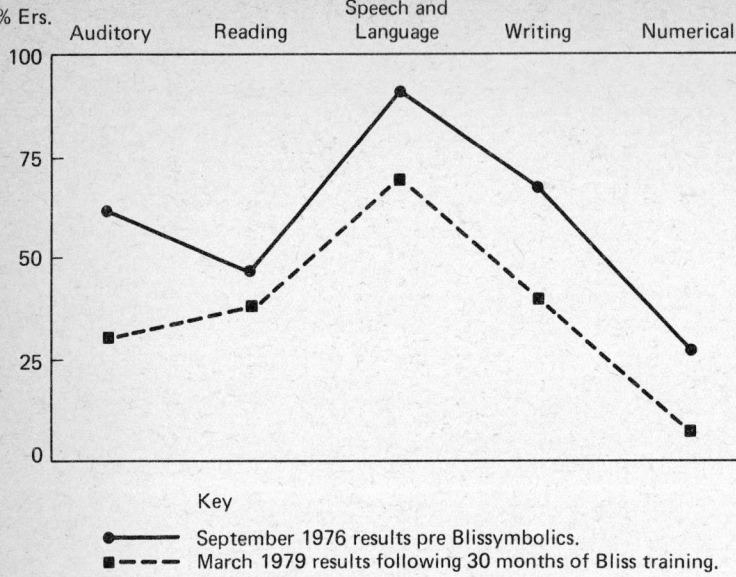

Figure 16.1 Change in MTDDA scores during Bliss programme

improvement all occurred more than 9 MPO, after extensive natural-language therapy. It is therefore unlikely to be solely attributable to spontaneous recovery.

A comparison of change in verbal and nonverbal test scores illustrates the consistently superior nonverbal skills (See Figure 16.2). The slight decline in RSPM scores is not unusual in dysphasic patients and occurs with the coloured as well as standard versions of the test. A possible explanation may be that right-hemisphere language is responsible for some of the early recovery in dysphasia thus reducing the functional capacity of the right hemisphere for dealing with nonverbal material. B.L. scored 100 per cent on the RCPM at the initial administration. For this reason the RSPM was used thereafter. Saya (1979) found that in his group of 10 dysphasics better scores on RCPM correlated positively with better Bliss-symbol acquisition. The only other two subjects for whom Blissymbols were thought to be a possible alternative both demonstrated some difficulty with RCPM and failed to progress beyond the symbol-matching level.

Although Koh's Block Design Test is also a nonverbal test it has been found that dysphasics capable of a reasonable performance on the Matrices may be unable to cope with block design, in the absence of any other evidence of a parietal dysfunction. Again B.L.'s initial performance was better than that achieved by the majority of dysphasics, including those with functional use of both hands.

After a three and a half year trial of the system it would appear that Bliss was probably not an ideal alternative communication system for B.L. but it had proved to be a valuable treatment technique. The reason may be that a programme designed to stimulate language development and communication in children cannot be equally effective in the adult whose problem is a breakdown in language

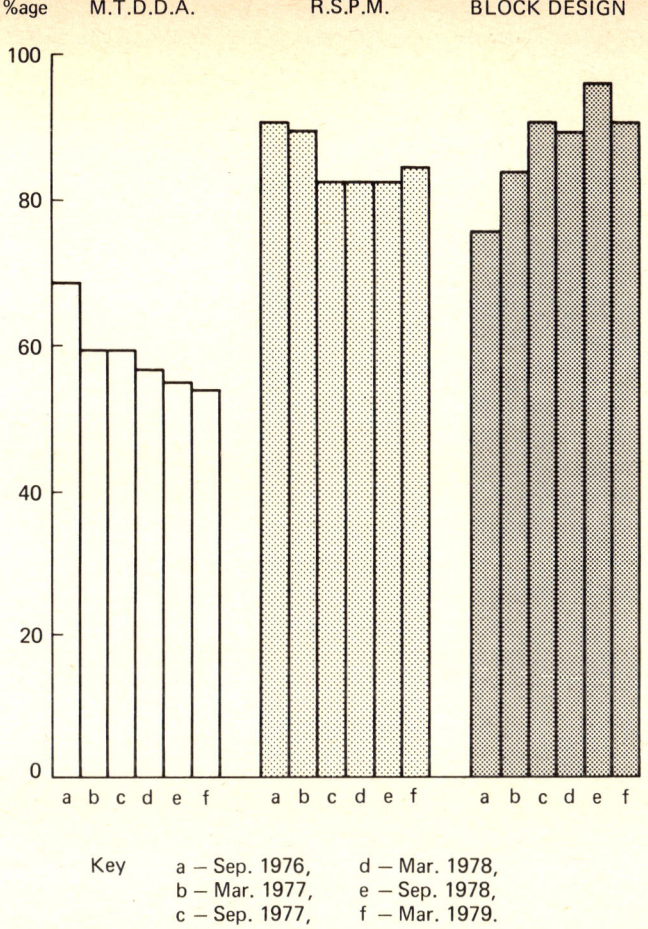

Figure 16.2 Change in verbal and non-verbal test performances during Bliss programme (MTDDA are percentage error scores).

retrieval. There is amongst aphasic patients generally a great reluctance to adopt any 'unnatural' method of communication. Saya (1979) comments that his best symbol learner would only use symbols to communicate as a last resort. Ross (1979) found a similar reluctance in her experience of using Blissymbols with a 14-year-old who had sustained a head injury resulting in dysphasia, and her view that symbols 'must be modified to accommodate the needs of an adult who has the particular problems due to brain damage and symbol use should be integrated with other means of communication available' (p. 108), is supported by the experience with B.L.

Teaching Bliss it soon became clear that any aspect of the system which requires a degree of adjustment by the instructor is likely to produce a problem for the dysphasic who, as a result of brain damage, is less able to adapt than the normal adult. The previous experience with normal communication is also significant. Like Ross's subject, B.L. did not easily accept the simplified grammar; both preferred to write in omitted words.

The demonstrable improvement in B.L.'s language is a very positive encouragement for the use of Blissymbols with dysphasic adults. Why and how it was effective is important for future patient selection. One of the major factors in introducing symbols had been his apparently good right-hemisphere function. There was no information as to the degree of lateralization of language function in B.L. pre-trauma; however the high degree of skill that he has developed in using his left hand suggest a greater flexibility than is normally encountered in normal right-handers. B.L.'s sister and aunt were reported as being left-handed, and it has been suggested that familial sinistrality is associated with less dependance on left-hemisphere language function (Searleman 1977). Could B.L.'s partial recovery be due to right-hemisphere language?

An attempt to investigate the possible extent of right-hemisphere involvement in B.L.'s limited language recovery was initiated by measuring his visual field preference (VFP). The results could, of course, only be of limited value as this investigation was not undertaken before the Bliss programme was initiated; they were however interesting as they demonstrated a strong left VFP for both verbal and nonverbal material. The brain scan initiated by these findings confirmed that the major part of what are generally regarded as the language areas had been affected and therefore suggested that their role in his present language skills must be limited. Clearly it would be valuable to have information on VFP before any Bliss programme was initiated with other subjects in the future.

Conclusion

The original hope, that relieving frustration might alleviate the articulatory dyspraxia, was not fulfilled. Although there has been evidence of some intelligible single-word utterances this is not consistent or reliable. B.L. has however objectively and functionally improved his communicative skill and understanding of language.

As a result of their investigation Moore and Weidner (1974) concluded that 'methods which afford greater linguistic stimulation of the right hemisphere may reduce the amount of time in active therapy, (p. 1010). It is much too premature to claim that Blissymbolics may be such a method, but the results of this trial would seem to encourage further investigation and more widespread use of Bliss with selected patients as an alternative treatment technique.

17

Communication aid and therapeutic tool: a report on the clinical trial using SPLINK with aphasic patients

Pam Enderby and Guy Hamilton

Introduction

It is evident that evaluation of communication aids in a functional situation is a necessary part of their development, because of the various social, psychological and practical factors related to their acceptability. This is indicated by many unexpected findings in the trial results of one such aid, 'Splink', presented here. This multi-centre trial studied 127 subjects with a variety of speech and language disabilities that limited spontaneous conversation. The results that are detailed in this paper refer to 37 of these patients diagnosed as aphasic, who were examined as a sub-group in the trial. The results indicate that a substantial number of these patients would benefit from using this aid as a communicator and/or a therapeutic tool.

A clinical trial is the only way of establishing the value and versatility of a communication aid, so that useful future comparisons with other systems may be made. This Splink trial has concerned itself with situations where the aid may be of benefit and with comparisons of individual communicative ability with the aid and without it.

The word Splink is derived from 'Speech Link'. The device gives the user direct access to a small, manageable electronic word-board, consisting of 950 basic words, letters of the alphabet, numerals, common phrases and various prefixes and suffixes along with instruction controls which increase its versatility (see Figure 17.1). The lap-sized, wire-less word-board transmits by infra-red to a microprocessor box which is plugged into the aerial socket of any unmodified television set so that when the words on the word-board are depressed, they appear on the television screen. The words can be sequenced into sentences and corrections can be made. The infra-red feature gives the user mobility, with no wires to trail inconveniently, within 12 to 15 feet between board and the television set (see Figure 17.2). Two or more word-boards may transmit to the single microprocessor and television set enabling groups of users to communicate with each other.

An initial trial (Enderby and Hamilton 1979) was carried out using three prototype Splinks. This trial was designed to gauge its *usefulness* as a sole communicator, as an aid to communication and as a teaching aid; to establish the aid's *acceptability* to patients, staff and public; to investigate its *practicality*, reliability, durability and versatility; and to define the *capability* of different groups of patients to use Splink. The results of this trial suggested that this aid may be useful for patients with language disorders as well as the speech disorders for which it was

188   ALTERNATIVE COMMUNICATION METHODS

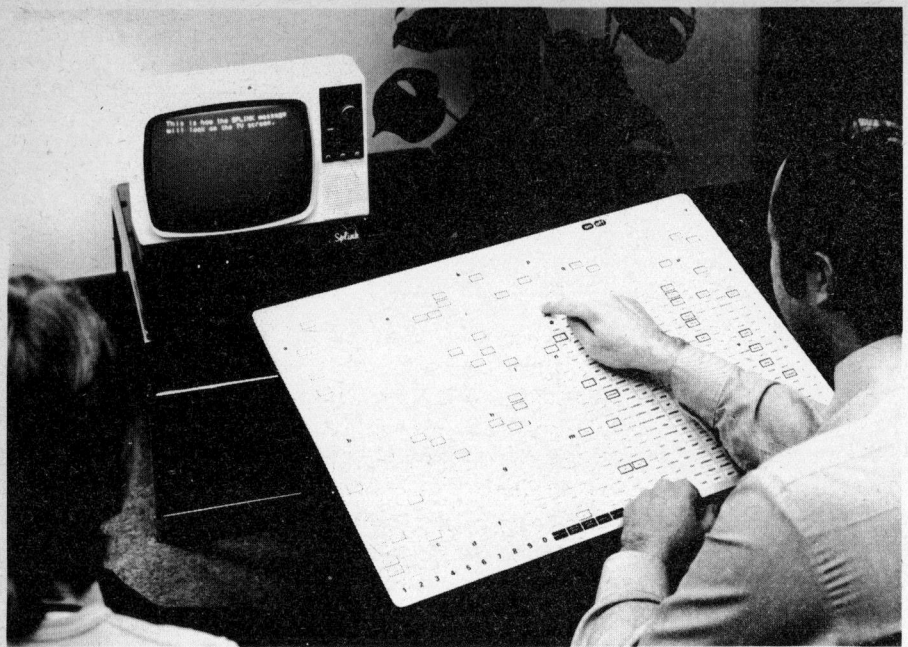

Figure 17.1 Splink in use.

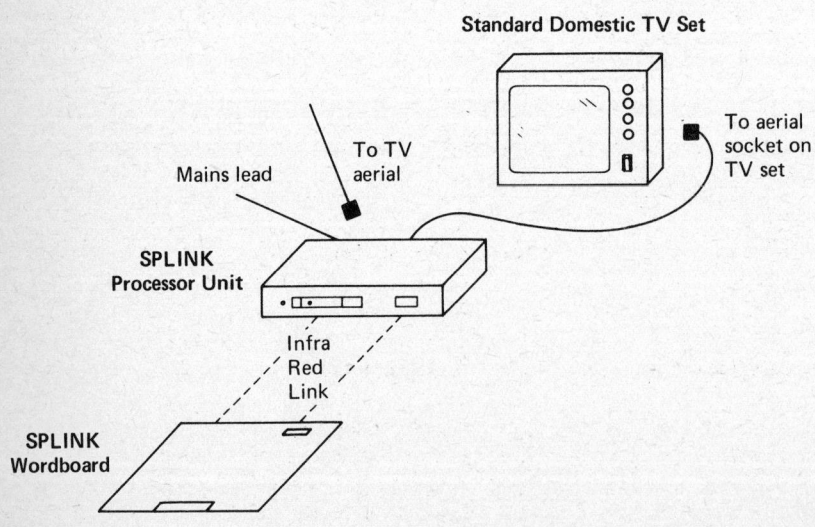

Figure 17.2 The Splink system.

designed. This study of 20 patients indicated the necessity for a larger-scale trial to examine in detail responses of different patient groups.

The multi-centre trial (Enderby and Hamilton 1981) incorporated some practical modifications, and additionally the methodology of the trial was changed to incorporate more information from therapists, teachers and relatives concerned, as the importance of their attitudes cannot be over-emphasized and it appears that the opinions of these people are as important as the patients themselves.

Method

Forty units were produced incorporating the necessary modifications and distributed to 29 centres in the United States of America and the United Kingdom. Valid responses were obtained from 19, which included 4 special schools, 10 district hospitals and 5 special units. Each centre had one or more units for at least 3 months. Guidelines were issued to all the centres taking part in the trial to ensure that similar relevant information was gathered on each subject. For instance, the method of introducing this aid to a patient was described as well as a suggestion that a patient should try the aid for a period of a fortnight before the results were assessed. Despite this, it was not surprising that the practical and philosophical approaches of various centres made it difficult to obtain comparable data. However, the different approaches in themselves have taught us a great deal about the use of aids in general.

Subjects

The 37 aphasic patients were selected by therapists as probably being physically, visually and linguistically capable of using Splink. Details of 107 patients with a variety of speech handicaps examined in this trial are also available (Enderby and Hamilton, 1981). The medical aetiology and method of communication of all subjects is shown in Table 17.1.

Table 17.1 The medical aetiology, degree of physical handicap and method of communication of all subjects.

Medical	Cerebral vascular accident	26
	Cerebral aneurysms	4
	Subarachnoid haemorrhage	3
	Myocardial infarction	2
	Unknown	2
Physical handicap	Right hemiplegia	29
	Left hemiplegia	3
	No physical handicap	5
Present method of communication	No method of communication	14
	One-word utterances and/or gesture	16
	Other assistive device (mostly pointing boards)	4
	Verbal communication with difficulty	3

The mean age was 59 years with a range between 33 and 71 years. Eighteen subjects were female and 19 male. All patients were diagnosed by a speech therapist as being dysphasic. In addition, nine patients had a secondary speech impairment of dysarthria and/or dyspraxia.

Thirty patients used the aid in the clinical situation with the therapist, volunteer or relative. Of these 30, nine also took the aid to be used in the home. Seven patients used Splink at home only. Twenty-nine patients had a right hemiplegia, three had a left hemiplegia and five had no physical handicap.

Splink was loaned to patients for a minimum period before the results form was completed. It was necessary that patients and relatives should have this time to become accustomed to the aid. Additionally, this length of time acknowledges the possibility of a 'novelty' factor which should be taken into account.

Results

Patients, therapists and relatives were questioned with regard to the use of Splink over the trial period. Nine patients found Splink useful in communication, 12 patients used Splink as an extension to therapy, 3 patients were more fully assessed using Splink and 13 patients were unable to use the aid. Of the 12 patients using it as an extension to therapy, but unable to use it spontaneously, eight had previously been unable to do any home practise of language tasks because of severe perseveration or dysgraphia. Splink enabled them to perform tasks set by the therapists on their own, for example such tasks as copying, word-finding and sentence completion. In addition, the interest generated by using an electronic 'gadget' appeared to encourage patients to persist with otherwise rather repetitive tasks.

The majority of these patients have used the Splink as a therapeutic tool in a structured situation. The seven patients with associated dyspraxia had greater success in using it to expand spontaneous communication; five of these were reported by relatives as having improved spoken output during the trial. This could probably be explained by reduced stress in both patients and relatives, facilitating oral control.

Included in the 13 patients who could not use Splink were 10 who had more severe lexic, linguistic and organizational problems than were previously recognized by the therapist involved. The combinations of disorders found in this population can make it difficult to determine which is predominantly more handicapping. In this group there were three patients who showed little interest in using the aid and were reported to have little motivation or initiative. This was despite the fact that they were able to express basic wants and needs via this medium when prompted and encouraged. This lack of spontaneity and initiative had not been noticed by the aphasia therapist previously, but obviously was important to recognize with regard to planning future management of their care.

The nine patients who used Splink as a communicator as well as a therapy tool showed great deal of interest in the aid itself, and tended to use it spontaneously to initiate an idea, but all used it telegrammatically. This abbreviated language structure could be due to linguistic disability, impaired visual memory, difficulty in selection of the appropriate words. There was not one patient in the aphasic group who could use this device without a great deal of guidance and encouragement. This is unlike the patients studied in the other non-aphasic groups, who demonstrated variability in the necessity and extent of training required.

The majority of relatives, or in three cases, the care staff, were interested in Splink. However, many were worried about whether it could be broken and anxious about caring for the aid. Support and encouragement of the relative by the therapist seemed necessary initially. In two cases the aid was not used at home by the patient due to anxiety on the part of the spouse which resulted in the Splink being carefully stored away. The suspicion of some patients and relatives could be related to age—the younger family being able to accommodate to technology more easily.

Of the 21 patients who could use Splink, all finally reported that they 'liked it'. This was despite the initial statements that they were overawed and perplexed, and in fact, not one subject in this group showed immediate potential when faced with Splink. Therapists working with dysphasic patients are fully aware that there are no simple answers, and it is therefore surprising that some would prematurely desist with this technical appliance when initial responses were disappointing. It is possible that therapists who are trained to be flexible in their approach and to minimize patient failure are being counter-productive in some spheres. The necessity for very patient repetitive training to teach a brain-damaged adult to adapt to a new concept of communication in addition to overcoming the practical and social difficulties which may be encountered in a home housing an aid, *cannot be underestimated*.

Therapeutic applications

Therapists involved in the trial reported certain tasks could be performed with Splink by some patients. These tasks included copying of sentences, sentence completion, word-finding, picture description, sequencing, spelling, recognition and initiation of functor words. Many of the aphasic patients did not require the size of vocabulary available as some words were beyond their range of competence. Several therapists and patients commented that they would have preferred a board with a smaller vocabulary to ease scanning and to speed up accessing of words. This recommendation has been passed on to the manufacturer. In the interim, some therapists have designed 'masks' which only expose the words that they wish to work with. These masks can be altered to expose more words as the patient becomes ready to assimilate more. A colour-coding system can be used to facilitate location of certain words. This colour-coding can be changed according to the method being used with the patient; some patients find it helpful, for instance, to have nouns and verbs identified by different colours. With other patients, the words that they use most frequently or are particularly pertinent to their environment can be identified by colour. There has also been success with colour identifying certain difficult parts of speech, such as prepositions, which have been otherwise omitted. It appears that there are many patients who are reluctant to work upon linguistic exercises at home because of their verbal or graphic disabilities which embarrass them. Some of these patients have been able to practice exercises given by the therapist with greater ease and therefore have persisted for longer. It is interesting that the 'TV game' aspect of Splink has resulted in patients pursuing conventional speech-therapy tasks with a new persistent vigour. If we are concerned with regard to increasing the amount of therapy a patient receives, any method which encourages the dysphasic patient to 'treat' him or herself is worth serious consideration.

Discussion

It is possible that patients who have to grapple with overcoming their oral and/or graphic disabilities are unable to directly access their linguistic competence and develop their linguistic capabilities. It has been shown that comprehension and reading often demonstrate more extensive spontaneous recovery (Kertesz and McCabe 1977) and this could be one of the reasons why Splink has been demonstrated to be of value to some dysphasic patients. This initiates a new therapeutic concept of tapping receptive abilities as an expressive mode. There are several non-speech communication methods (Goldstein and Cameron 1952; Eagleson, Vaughn and Knudson 1970; Glass, Gazzaniga and Premack 1973; Schlanger 1976) which have been used with dysphasic patients and all suggest that there is a direct positive effect on verbal expression. 'Success with this non-speech mode of communication increased the apparent motivation of patients to persevere in learning verbal modes of communication' (Eagleson *et al*. 1970, 112).

Silverman (1980) supports the view that non-speech communication modes can be used with dysphasic patients on a temporary or permanent basis to facilitate communication. 'Those with moderate to severe deficits in speech comprehension, speaking, reading and writing may be able to communicate basic needs to persons taking care of them by pointing—pantomiming, or by using manual sign language' (p. 7). The needs for such communication modes may be permanent or temporary. Silverman continues to present some evidence which suggests that non-speech communication modes used during the immediate post-trauma period may facilitate recovery.

Splink was not developed with the aphasic population in mind and it is interesting and exciting to find that imaginative use of an aid can increase its versatility. It is too easy to assume that the increasing number of communication aids will immediately and of themselves alleviate the plight of some speech-handicapped patients and it is necessary for aphasia therapists to be aware of developments in related fields and examine their applicability without prejudice.

Aphasia Therapy Research: A Single-Case Study Approach

In this concluding chapter, Coltheart discusses the single-case study approach to evaluating the ongoing effectiveness of specific techniques in therapy. This method of testing the outcome of treatment emphasizes that the experimental study of individual behaviour can be of more relevance to the aphasia therapist than larger-scale studies. This may point to a future role for the clinician as both therapist and researcher and help bridge the gap between theory and practice. Some of the problems of the large-scale study approach are discussed by David in chapter 2.

18

Aphasia therapy research: a single-case study approach

Max Coltheart

It will be assumed that the main aim of aphasia therapy is as stated explicitly in chapter 2 by David:

> to improve the quality of the patient's life by increasing communicative ability.

There may, of course, be other ways in which one could attempt to improve the quality of the aphasic patient's life—by dealing with interpersonal and family problems caused only indirectly by aphasia, as discussed in chapter 8 by Müller and Code, or by considering the effects of aphasia upon a patient's personality and self-concept, as discussed in chapter 7 by Brumfitt and Clarke—but such issues are as much the province of the social worker or clinical psychologist as of the speech therapist, and will not be considered further here. Instead this chapter will be concerned solely with the aphasia therapist's attempts to improve a patient's ability to communicate with those around him or her and to understand their communications.

As this volume demonstrates, there is no shortage of ideas about ways in which the aphasia therapist might set about treating any of the various linguistic impairments shown by aphasic patients. Such ideas may involve technical aids, as discussed in the chapters by Rowley (15) and by Enderby and Hamilton (17); they may involve artificial communication systems such as Blissymbolics (discussed by Bailey, chapter 16) or VIC (discussed by Rowley, chapter 15); a radical approach involving contributions to language from the right hemisphere is considered in Code's chapter (4); and other chapters proffer other ideas. What there *is* a drastic shortage of is evidence concerning the degree to which any of these, or any other, techniques *do* improve the aphasic's communicative capacities. Research on the efficacy of aphasia therapy is still at a primitive stage, and few if any of the published efficacy studies are free from serious methodological difficulties.

Let us suppose that there are treatment methods which if used would genuinely improve the linguistic capabilities of the aphasic patient—even if we do not yet know what these methods are, nor how to demonstrate their genuine effectiveness. If such treatment methods do exist, then the ultimate goal of the speech-therapy profession must be to bring about a situation in which these methods are in standard use in speech-therapy clinics. For this to occur, it is not enough for an appropriate method to be discovered by some individual. What would be needed is a demonstration of efficacy which is convincing to other members of the profession—and which is disseminated in a way which allows it to become public knowledge. If this is so, then surely the future progress of aphasia therapy will depend crucially upon methodologically adequate studies of efficacy being conducted, and their results published. In this chapter some suggestions as to how one might go about designing and executing such studies are made. These suggestions are intended to be practical ones, in the sense that the amount of additional effort needed to transform normal clinical work into methodologically acceptable research would appear to be not very great. That is, if the therapeutic work is going to occur anyway, then with a little prior reflection and preparation the therapist can collect data in the course of normal therapeutic work which will provide information concerning the effectiveness of the therapy.

Patient description

The first step is to compile a description of the patient's aphasic symptomatology. This might include scores on a standardized aphasia test battery, but therapists' descriptions of the ways in which the patient's language is disordered would seem to be indispensable. The point of putting together this description is as follows. Suppose that the particular therapeutic methods used with the patient were successful. If efficacy research is to be a cumulative endeavour, one would expect further research work on these methods. This work could be replication, i.e., exact repetition of the original research; and to carry out an exact repetition one would need to study a similar kind of patient. This could only be done if a sufficiently detailed description of the original patient were available. Alternatively, the future research might be an extension of the original research—for example, it might seek to discover whether the same treatment method would be successful with a *different* kind of patient. Here again one needs a satisfactory description of the original patient in order to know what would count as a different kind of patient.

Patient description is also important if the outcome of the original efficacy study is negative, i.e., yielded evidence suggesting that the particular therapeutic methods used do not lead to improvement. If these methods are widely used ones, or if they appear to be particularly plausible, one might not wish to discard them on the basis of a single patient's response to them: so here exact replication would again be desirable. Alternatively, one might want to investigate whether these methods might be effective with other types of patient. In either case, to be able to carry out the follow-up research one would need to have available a good description of the original patient's linguistic impairments. Thus any study intending to obtain information about the efficacy of any form of treatment should begin with the assembling of a good description of the patient.

Defining the function or functions to be treated

The next step is to decide upon and to define the particular aspects of the patient's disordered language which are to be the object of the treatment. What is of essence here is to avoid being too general whilst also avoiding being too specific. A decision to treat the patient's speech would be too general. Would this mean speech perception or speech production? If speech production, would it mean improving articulation, or increasing the use of function words in spontaneous speech, or dealing with a disorder of intonation? A too general definition of this kind provides an inadequate focus for devising specific therapeutic regimes, and poses insuperable problems concerning how the patient's linguistic functioning should be measured.

On the other hand, it is possible to be too specific. If one defined the linguistic function to be treated as the ability to produce stop consonants, and the patient in question were a Broca's aphasic with a difficulty in producing such consonants, it is unlikely that an improvement in this highly specific function would contribute much to improving the patient's ability to communicate with others, since speech would continue to be syntactically impoverished.

To illustrate the level of specificity of linguistic functioning envisaged, here are some examples of linguistic functions defined at a useful level of specificity:

(a) Spelling.
(b) Using function words in spontaneous speech.
(c) Nonverbal behaviour assisting conversational speech.
(d) Reading isolated words aloud.
(e) Naming pictures and objects.
(f) Speech comprehension at the single-sentence level.
(g) Lip-reading.
(h) Reading comprehension at the paragraph level.

These are all functions which, if impaired, could have quite severe consequences for a patient, and which therefore are important enough to deserve treatment; at the same time all of these functions are specific enough that one can think in concrete terms about methods of treatment and about how to devise methods of measuring how well the patient can perform the function.

Once a description of the patient has been formulated, as advocated earlier, one can then list some of the linguistic functions in which there is impairment, and then select from these one or more which are to be treated.

Measurement

If the treatment is to be carried out in the context of an efficacy study, then before-and-after measurement is required. Hence, once a decision has been made concerning which functions are to be treated, one then has to decide how this function is to be measured. Here it is rarely the case that one can turn to already existing tests: often no relevant test exists, and where there are relevant tests available they are usually much too unsophisticated and, more importantly, contain far too few items to allow sufficient precision of measurement. Thus it is often necessary to construct new measurement methods. In practice this is usually not difficult: and this is one of the stages of efficacy research where the experimental psychologist or the linguist can often make useful contributions. For example, if the therapist wishes to measure picture-naming ability, a large pool of pictures with unambiguous names may be needed: such a pool has recently been collected, tested and published by psychologists (Snodgrass and Vandervart 1980). Selection of stimulus material by computer is now possible: the MRC Psycholinguistic Database (Coltheart 1981b) consists of more than 98,000 words stored on file in a computer, with a great deal of orthographic, phonological and semantic information about these words. This database could be used, for example, to select large lists of common monosyllabic five-letter abstract nouns, if therapeutic plans involved treating the ability to deal with this particular kind of word: or polysyllabic words could be selected containing consonant clusters, which might be useful for measuring dyspraxic difficulty in speech.

If the definitions of linguistic function decided upon are sufficiently specific, this greatly simplifies the development of measurement methods. As an illustration, here are examples of ways of measuring the eight functions listed above:

(a) Spelling: here it is simply a question of compiling in advance a sufficiently large set of words to allow selection of different random samples of words for each measurement occasion (if one wants to avoid practice effects by using no word more than once).

(b) Use of function words in spontaneous speech: one thing which is likely to be important here is to have control over the stimulus used to evoke speech. A conversational situation is not sufficiently controlled: different conversations might themselves evoke function words to different degrees. Picture-description, as used in the Boston (Goodglass and Kaplan 1972) and Whurr (1974) aphasia batteries, appears to be a useful method. Thus a large enough number of adequately complicated pictures are selected, and the patient is asked to describe a set of these on each measurement occasion. The spoken output thus evoked can then be scored for the presence of function words. There are many other ways of approaching this measurement issue, of course: just one example has been given.

(c) Nonverbal behaviour assisting conversation: a typical way of measuring this would be to have several people converse with the patient, and to ask them to rate the adequacy of nonverbal behaviour relevant to the conversation. Rating reliability can be assessed by determining how well the various raters agree with each other. Ratings of this sort need to be carried out blind, of course—that is, the raters do not know at what stage of treatment the patient is.

(d) Reading isolated words aloud: this, like the testing of spelling, requires the prior availability of a large enough set of stimulus words. If one is interested in the patient's ability to read certain kinds of words—abstract words, for example, or function words—then there will be restrictions on the kinds of words one selects and here the psycholinguistic database referred to above (Coltheart 1981b) is especially useful, since it can provide lists of words having the required properties. This saves a great deal of time, since drawing up lists of words which must meet prespecified criteria can otherwise be extremely time-consuming.

(e) Picture-naming: as already mentioned, the paper by Snodgrass and Vandervart (1980) is an invaluable source of stimuli for measuring the ability to name pictures.

(f) Speech comprehension at the sentence level: the Token Test (De Renzi and Vignolo 1962) is often used here. Whether this is appropriate depends upon whether one wants to measure the ability to understand extremely non-redundant sentences spoken without such normally occurring aids to comprehension as context and intonation, or whether one wants to measure sentence comprehension in a more naturalistic setting. If the latter, a new form of testing would be required

—conceivably even the rating by observers of a patient's ability to comprehend sentences in a conversational setting.

(g) Lip-reading: many aphasic patients appear to rely quite heavily upon lip-reading to circumvent as much as possible difficulties with the auditory comprehension of speech. This is not surprising since lip-reading plays some part in speech comprehension for the normal listener. The extent to which the aphasic patient relies upon lip-reading to identify spoken words can be assessed by comparing the ability to repeat heard words when the speaker's face is visible to the ability at this task when the eyes are shut. In conduction aphasia, repetition can be dramatically worse in the latter condition. Improvements in lip-reading ability can be measured as improvements in repetition ability with the speaker's face seen relative to repetition ability with the face unseen—or indeed lip-reading ability can be directly measured by presenting silently speaking faces (on videotape, for example, with the sound turned off).

(h) Reading comprehension at the paragraph level: here standardized tests may be useful, since there are a number which take the form of a paragraph followed by multiple-choice tests of comprehension. If insufficient material of this form is available, additional paragraphs and multiple-choice questions can be selected.

Measurement methods have been considered in such detail here in order to try to emphasize the fact that the *ad hoc* construction of new methods of measurement, and the eschewal of well known already existing standardized tests, is neither difficult nor unscientific: indeed what results is very often far more useful for scientific purposes than the well known tests. *Ad hoc* testing methods are, of course, not standardized, but standardization is irrelevant in individual case studies involving before-and-after measurement: the patient is not being compared with some control group, but with him or herself.

Treatment

The patient having been described, the linguistic functions to be treated having been defined, and the methods of measuring these functions having been decided upon, one can then proceed with treatment. As indicated earlier, there is no shortage amongst aphasia therapists of ideas about possible treatment methods: many of the chapters in this volume attest to that. However, the conviction expressed by Hatfield and Shewell in their chapter (5) is echoed here with fervour: that one is much more likely to discover effective treatment methods if one concentrates upon methods which are both *rational* (that is, based upon some theory of how the linguistic function concerned is normally performed) and *specific* (that is, adapted to the nature of the particular linguistic disorder exhibited). The programme for treating agrammatism which is set out in their chapter is one example of a rational and specific method of treatment. Further examples of rationality and specificity of treatment methods are evident in the chapter by Hatfield (14) dealing with the treatment of disorders of spelling.

If one's treatment is to be part of an efficacy study, then an additional requirement is that it be described in sufficient detail to allow it to be exactly duplicated by other therapists treating of other patients. This is obviously essential if further investigation of the treatment method is to be undertaken by others—or, indeed, if the treatment method has been successful enough to lead other therapists to wish to adopt it as standard practice. Ideally, the description of the method should be such that it would allow a non-specialist such as a volunteer or a member of the patient's family to carry out the treatment appropriately. If the aphasia therapist's job consisted mainly of inventing and testing treatment methods, and if the administration of treatment could be largely the job of non-specialists instructed by therapists, then of course the amount of treatment patients receive would be greatly increased.

Experimental design

The essence of efficacy research is to design studies in such a way as to allow one to determine whether or not any improvements in the patient's linguistic capabilities were *caused* by the specific treatment adopted, rather than being due to some non-specific effect of treatment (a general increase in motivation, for example) or to some factor entirely unrelated to treatment (spontaneous recovery, for example). If one simply measured the to-be-treated function before and after treatment and found that it was significantly improved after treatment, one could not demonstrate that this improvement was caused by the specific treatment method used.

In principle, one can overcome these difficulties with a group study in which three exactly comparable groups of patients are assigned to three conditions: treatment A, treatment B, and no treatment. If the no-treatment group do not improve, then spontaneous recovery is not occurring in this group, and since the three groups are exactly comparable, there is no spontaneous recovery occurring in the other two groups either. Therefore any improvement is due to treatment. If the treatment A group shows improvement whilst the treatment group B do not, it is reasonable to conclude that this improvement is a specific treatment effect.

In practice, the difficulties with this kind of experimental design are enormous. The interpretation of results from this design rests entirely on the exact comparability of the three groups prior to treatment. This comparability can be sought either by matching or by randomization. Matching consists of deliberately assigning patients to groups. Even if all the variables on which such matching should be done are known, adequate matching is probably impossible because there are too many variables likely to be correlated with prospects for recovery; and matching on even a few variables is clearly very difficult to achieve in practice, since no efficacy study appears to have been published in which adequate matching in all of the obvious major variables (age, sex, aetiology, time since onset, severity, premorbid educational level and aphasia type) has even been approximately achieved.

In addition, there are the ethical difficulties associated with a no-treatment condition. If the patients in this condition are untreated for a reason other than the research worker's decision (for example, if they are patients who *happen* not to have received treatment because, for example, they live in an isolated region, or because they refused treatment) then the comparability of this group to the treatment groups has been lost, and hence the no-treatment group can no longer contribute validly to the experimental design. If, on the other hand, patients are assigned to the no-treatment group, deliberately (via matching) or not (via randomization), by the research worker, then these are patients who, if they had not participated in the efficacy study, might otherwise have received treatment.

These problems for the group-study approach, and others such as those described by Darley (1972b) and Lapointe (1978), are, it is suggested, effectively insurmountable; it is argued here that, not only have no unambiguous conclusions concerning the efficacy of any form of aphasia therapy emerged from any of the group studies so far undertaken, but that any such studies in the future will be no more successful. The claim made here is that the methodological difficulties can only be circumvented by longitudinal single-case studies (or, what is equivalent, studies which use a small number of patients exhibiting a homogeneous symptomatology and in which the response of each patient to the treatment may be studied —such studies are effectively *sets* of individual case studies).

The matching problem is dealt with by comparing patients with themselves. There are a number of ways of dealing with the problem of spontaneous recovery. One is to withhold treatment for periods. For example, one can measure the to-be-treated function at intervals prior to beginning treatment: if it does not improve during this period, but does improve during treatment, spontaneous recovery could hardly be the evaluation. However, the ethical problem remains. It can be avoided with a different kind of experimental design, which might be called the *crossover-treatment* design.

This design requires one to select at least two linguistic functions for treatment. Suppose exactly two are selected: call them X and Y. Prior to treatment, the patient's ability to perform both X and Y is measured (Test 1). Then there follows a period of treatment: but only one function is treated (let us say X). At the end of this period both functions are re-tested (Test 2). Then there follows a period during which only Y is treated. Finally, both functions are re-tested again (Test 3).

If function X is no better in Test 2 than Test 1 then the treatment of X has been ineffective. If function Y is no better in Test 3 than Test 2 then the treatment of Y has been ineffective.

Suppose X *is* better at Test 2 than Test 1. If this is just due to spontaneous recovery and has nothing to do with X having been treated, one would expect the *untreated* function, Y, also to have improved: hence if X improves more than Y over the period from Test 1 to Test 2, this is evidence for a specific treatment effect. One might object to this inference by arguing that perhaps X happens to be a function which tends to improve more, spontaneously, than Y. There are two ways of rebutting this argument. The first is to repeat the study with another patient but this time treat Y before X. The second is to look at what happens between Test 2 and Test 3. If during this period X does not improve whilst Y does (whereas in the period between Test 1 and Test 2 X improved and Y did not) then explanations in terms of spontaneous recovery become untenable.

This design also allows one to test for the *permanence* of treatment effects, something which is essential for any efficacy study. Clearly, improvements which last for very short periods of time are of little importance—and one does find such ephemeral improvements. Chapter 6, by Patterson, Purell and Morton includes a demonstration that the facilitation of object-naming which can be achieved by repetition or phonemic cueing persists for less than half an hour. In the crossover-treatment design, the permanence of any improvements in function X can be determined by comparing performance on this function at Test 2 with performance at Test 3. If one wishes to assess the permanence of any improvements in the function treated second (Y), then a further test is needed: if there is a period after Test 3 during which Y is not treated, one can re-test Y after this no-treatment period to see if the improvements have persisted.

Investigating *generalizability* is also important, and can be accomplished using this design. Let us suppose function X is reading aloud isolated words. If a patient is given repeated practice in reading aloud a fixed set of words, and if success rate does improve, it is necessary to know whether the patient has learned something specific about this particular set of words, of something more general about how to read *any* set of words. Within the crossover-treatment design this is accomplished as follows. Suppose a set of 80 words is selected and administered in the pre-test phase (Test 1). Half of these words are chosen and used during the treatment phase; the other half are never seen by the patient during this phase. Then all 80 are administered at the Test 2 (post-treatment) stage. A generalized effect on reading is indexed by the Test 2 *vs* Test 1 difference in performance with the words *not* used during treatment; effects due to specific experience with particular words during treatment are indexed by what happens between Test 1 and Test 2 to the words which *were* used during treatment.

Although it would be somewhat disappointing to find that a treatment effect is material-specific—that, for example, a patient's improvements in reading aloud are confined to those particular words on which there has been training and do not generalize to other words—such material-specific effects are not trivial. Their existence demonstrates that the patient can re-acquire some linguistic skills, even if only very specific ones; and limited re-acquisition of limited skills can make a difference to the patient's life. A patient who, having lost entirely the ability to recall the names of neighbours when their faces are seen, is slowly and specifically re-taught, say, 10 such names is obviously much better off as a consequence, even if the *general* ability to memorize has not been improved.

The crossover-treatment design is not entirely free of problems: there are possible outcomes of the design which are not immediately interpretable. For example suppose comparison of Test 1 with Test 2 showed that the treated function X and the untreated function Y had improved to the same extent. This could be spontaneous recovery; or it could be that the treatment of X actually assisted function Y as well, which could happen if X and Y were related functions (such as reading aloud and picture-naming). In the first case, there is no treatment effect; in the second case there is. Equal improvement of X and Y is thus an ambiguous outcome unless it is quite implausible that treating X should affect Y; which suggests that when one chooses the two functions one ought if possible to choose two very different functions, where treatment of one is very unlikely to affect the other.

If ambiguities of this kind do arise, they need to be dealt with by further work on other patients—possibly even by some assessment of whether functions X and Y do spontaneously improve prior to the beginning of treatment.

This kind of design does not seem to be open to objections on the grounds of the ethical difficulties associated with withholding treatment, because a patient taking part in this kind of study would receive just as much treatment as if he or she were not participating: the difference is that the treatment is distributed differently across time. Instead of getting a mixture of X and Y treatments across a period of n weeks, the patient gets all of the X treatment concentrated in the first half of the n-week period, and all of the Y treatment concentrated in the second half of this period.

Conclusions

It has been argued in this chapter that it is possible for the individual speech therapist to discover, and to demonstrate rigorously to colleagues, whether specific treatment regimes are or are not effective in alleviating specific aphasic symptoms. Efficacy research of this kind does not require investigations of large groups of aphasic subjects—indeed, it has been suggested that large-scale studies are less likely to be informative than the kind of individual case study that has been advocated above. Nor does such efficacy research require the collection of data unrelated to the normal clinical work of the aphasia therapist, since the data collection derives directly from this clinical work: measuring patients' linguistic performance is part of normal clinical practice. Ideas as to the treatment of aphasia abound; what is needed if aphasia therapy is to progress at all is for research into the efficacy of treatments based on these ideas to become much more common, and for the results of such research to be much more widely disseminated.

References

ADAMS, J.A. 1976: *Learning and memory*. Homewood, Illinois: The Dorsey Press.
AJAX, E.T. 1967: Dyslexia without agraphia: prognostic considerations. *Arch. Neurol.* **17**, 645–52.
AKHUTINA, T.V. 1978: Comprehension and production of active and passive structures by aphasic patients. In H. Mierzejewska (ed.), *Badana Lingwistyczne nad Afazja*. Warsaw: Ossolineum (in Russian).
ALBERT, M.L. and BEAR, D. 1974: Time to understand: a case study in word deafness with reference to the role of time in auditory comprehension. *Brain* **97**, 373–84.
ALBERT, M.L., SPARKS, R. and HELM, N. 1973: Melodic intonation therapy for aphasia. *Arch. Neurol.* **29**, 130–1.
ARGYLE, M. 1975: *Bodily communication*. New York: Cambridge University Press.
ARMSTRONG, D.M. 1976: *A materialist theory of the mind*. London: Routledge & Kegan Paul.
ARTES, R. and HOOPS, R. 1976: Problems of aphasic and non-aphasic stroke patients as identified and evaluated by patients' wives. In Y. Lebrun and R. Hoops (eds.), *Recovery in aphasics*. Amsterdam: Swets & Zeitlinger.
BAKER, E., BERRY, T., GARDNER, H., ZURIF, E., DAVIS, L. and VEROFF, A. 1975: Can linguistic competence be dissociated from natural language functions? *Nature* **254**, 509–10.
BANNISTER, D. and FRANSELLA, F. 1980: *Inquiring man. The theory of personal constructs* (2nd edn). Harmondsworth: Penguin.
BANNISTER, D. and MAIR, J.M.M. 1968: *The evaluation of personal constructs*. London: Academic Press.
BASSO, A., CAPITANI, E. and VIGNOLO, L.A. 1979: Influence of rehabilitation on language skills in aphasic patients: a controlled study. *Arch. Neurol.* **36**, 190–6.
BASSO, A., CASATI, G. and VIGNOLO, L.A. 1977: Phonemic identification defect in aphasia. *Cortex* **13**, 85–95.
BASSO, A., DE RENZI, E., FAGLIONI, P., SCOTTI, G. and SPINNLER, H. 1973: Neuropsychological evidence for the existence of cerebral areas critical to the performance of intellectual tests. *Brain* **96**, 715–28.
BASSO, A., FAGLIONI, P. and VIGNOLO, L. 1975: Étude controlée de la rééducation de language dans l'aphasie: comparaison entre aphasiques traités et non traités. *Review Neurologique* (Paris) **131**, 607–14.

BAY, E. 1964: Present concepts of aphasia. *Geriatrics* **19**, 319–31.
BEAUVOIS, M.F. and DÉROUESNÉ, J. 1981: Lexical or orthographic agraphia. *Brain* **104**, 21–49.
BECHTEREVA, N.P., BUNDZEN, P.V., GOGOLITSIN, Y.L., MALYSHEV, V.M. and PEREPELKIN, P.D. 1979: Neurophysiological codes or words in subcortical structures of the human brain. *Brain and Language* **7**, 145–63.
BENNETT, A.E. (ed.) 1976: *Communication between doctors and patients*. London: Nuffield Provincial Hospital Trust, Oxford University Press.
BENSON, D. 1977: The third alexia. *Arch. Neurol.* **34**, 327–31.
BERMAN, M. and PEELLE, L.M. 1967: Self-generated cues: a method for aiding aphasic and apraxic patients. *JSHD* **32**, 372–6.
BERNSTEIN, J.C. 1979: A supportive group for spouses of stroke patients. *Aphasia-Apraxia-Agnosia* **1**, 30–5.
BERNDT, R.S. and CARAMAZZA, A. 1980: A redefinition of the syndrome of Broca's aphasia: implications for a neuropsychological model of language. *Applied Psycholinguistics* **1**, 225–78.
BEYN, E.S. and SHOKHOR-TROTSKAYA, M.K. 1966: The preventive method of speech rehabilitation in aphasia. *Cortex* **2**, 96–108.
BINET, A., and SIMON, T. 1905: Méthodes nouvelles pour le diagnostic du niveau intellectuel des anormeaux. *L'Année Psychologique* **11**, 191–244.
BION, W.R. 1962: *Learning from experience*. London: Heinemann.
BISIACH, E. 1966: Perceptual factors in the pathogenesis of anomia. *Cortex* **11**, 90–5.
BLISS, C. 1965: *Semantography/Blissymbolics*. Sydney, Australia: Semantography Publications.
BLOOM, L.M. 1962: A rationale for group treatment of aphasic patients. *JSHD* **27**, 11–15.
BLUMSTEIN, S., BAKER, E. and GOODGLASS, H. 1977: Phonological factors in auditory comprehension in aphasia. *Neuropsychologia* **15**, 19–30.
BLUMSTEIN, S. and COOPER, W.E. 1974: Hemispheric processing of intonation contours. *Cortex* **10**, 146–57.
BOGEN, J.E. 1969: The other side of the brain II: an appositional mind. *Bulletin of the Los Angeles Neurological Societies* **34**, 135–62.
BOLLER, F., COLE, M., VRTUNSKI, P.B., PATTERSON, M. and KIM, Y. 1979: Paralinguistic aspects of auditory comprehension in aphasia. *Brain and Language* **7**, 164–74.
BOLLER, F., KIM, Y and MACK, J.L. 1977: Auditory comprehension in aphasia. In H. and H.A. Whitaker (eds.), *Studies in Neurolinguistics 3*. New York: Academic Press.
BOWLBY, J. 1980: *Attachment and loss. vol. III. Loss: sadness and depression*. London: Hogarth Press.
BOWLING, J.H. 1977: Emotional problems of relatives of dysphasic patients. *Aust. J. of Com. Dis.* **5**, 29–41.
BROCA, P. 1861: Nouvelle observation d'aphémie produite par une lésion de la moitié posterieure des deuxième et troisième circonvolutions frontales. *Bulletin de la Société Anatomique de Paris* **6**, 389–407.

BROCA, P. 1865: Sur le siege de la faculté du langage articulé. *Bulletin de la Société de'Anthropologie* **6**, 337–93.
BUFFERY, A.W. 1977: Clinical neuropsychology: a review and preview. In S. Rachman (ed.), *Contributions to medical psychology,* vol. 1. Oxford: Pergamon Press.
BUFFERY, A. and BURTON, A. (1982): Information-processing and redevelopment: towards a science of neuropsychological rehabilitation. In A. Burton (ed.), *The pathology and psychology of cognition*. London: Methuen.
BUCK, R. and DUFFY, R.J. 1980: Nonverbal communication of affect in brain damaged patients. *Cortex* **16**, 351–62.
BUCKINGHAM, H.W. 1979: Explanation in apraxia with consequences for the concept of apraxia of speech. *Brain and Language* **8**, 202–26.
BUTLER, S.R. and NORRSELL, U. 1968: Vocalization possibly initiated by the minor hemisphere. *Nature* **220**, 793–4.
CAMERON, J.A. 1976: *A proposal for research into visual communication systems for aphasia and related conditions*. Unpublished thesis in partial fulfilment of the MA degree in the Department of Visual Communication. Birmingham Polytechnic.
CARAMAZZA, A and BERNDT, R.S. 1978: Semantic and syntactic processes in aphasia: A review of the literature. *Psychological Bulletin* **85**, 898–918.
CASTRO-CALDAS, A. 1975: Experts and amateurs in stroke therapy. *The Lancet* **2** (7947), 1260.
CHOMSKY, N. 1957: *Syntactic structures*. The Hague: Mouton.
—— 1965: *Aspects of the theory of syntax*. Cambridge, Mass.: MIT Press.
CHRISTENSEN, A-L. 1974: *Luria's neuropsychological investigation: Text*. Copenhagen: Munksgaard.
CICONE, C., WAPNER, W. and GARDNER, H. 1980: Sensitivity to emotional expressions and situations in organic patients. *Cortex* **16**, 145–58.
CODE, C. 1981: Dichotic listening with the communicatively impaired. *J. of Phonetics* **9**, 375–83.
—— (1982): On the origins of recurrent utterances in aphasia. *Cortex* **18**, 161–64.
CODE, C. and BALL, M. (1982) Fricative production in Broca's aphasia: a spectography analysis. *J. of Phonetics* **10**, 325–31.
COHEN, G. 1977: *The psychology of cognition*. London: Academic Press.
COHEN, R. and KELTOR, S. 1979: Cognitive impairment of aphasics in a colour-to-picture matching task. *Cortex* **15**, 235–45.
COLTHEART, M. 1978: Lexical access in simple reading tasks. In G. Underwood, (ed.), *Strategies of information processing*. London: Academic Press.
—— 1980: Deep dyslexia: a right-hemisphere hypothesis. In M. Coltheart, K. Patterson and J.C. Marshall (eds.), *Deep dyslexia*. London: Routledge & Kegan Paul.
—— 1981b: The MRC psycholinguistic database. *Q. J. Exp. Psych.* **33a**, 497–506.
COLTHEART, M., PATTERSON, K. and MARSHALL, J.C. 1980: (eds.), *Deep Dyslexia*. London: Routledge & Kegan Paul.

COOK, M. 1979: *Perceiving others. The psychology of interpersonal perception*. London: Methuen.

CULTON, G.L. 1969: Spontaneous recovery from aphasia. *JSHR* **12**, 825–32.

CUMMINGS, J.L., BENSON, D.F., WALSH, M.J. and LEVINE, H.L. 1979: Left-to-right transfer of language dominance: a case study. *Neurology* **29**, 1547–50.

CRYSTAL, D., FLETCHER, P. and GARMAN, M. 1976: *The grammatical analysis of language disability*. London: Edward Arnold.

CZOPF, C. 1979: The role of the non-dominant hemisphere in speech recovery in aphasia. *Aphasia-Apraxia-Agnosia* **1**, 27–33.

DAMON, S., LESSER, R. and WOODS, R. 1979: Behavioural treatment of social difficulties with an aphasic woman and a dysarthric man. *BJDC* **14**, 31–8.

DANIELS, J.C. and DIACK, H. 1958: *The standard diagnostic tests of reading*. London: Chatto & Windus.

DARLEY, F.L. 1972a: The efficacy of language rehabilitation in aphasia. *JSHD* **30**, 3–22.

—— 1972b: Language rehabilitation in aphasia. *JSHD* **37**, 3–21.

DARLEY, F.L. 1975a: Current reviews of higher nervous system dysfunction. In W.J. Friedlander (ed.), *Advances in Neurology*, **7**. New York: Raven Press.

—— 1975b: Treatment of acquired aphasia. In W.J. Friedlander (ed.), *Advances in neurology, vol. 7. Current reviews of higher nervous system dysfunction*. New York: Raven Press.

DARLEY, F.L., ARONSON, A.E. and BROWN, J.R. 1975: *Motor speech disorders*. Philadelphia: Saunders.

DAVID, R.M. 1980: Interscorer reliability of the Functional Communication Profile. Unpublished data.

DAVID, R.M., ENDERBY, P. and BAINTON, D. 1979: Progress report on an evaluation of speech therapy for aphasia. *BJDC* **14**, 85–8.

DAVIS, L. and GARDNER, H. 1976: Strategies of mastering a visual communication system in aphasia. *Annals of New York Academy of Sciences* **280**, 885–97.

DAVIS, G.A. and WILCOX, M.J. 1981: Incorporating parameters of natural conversation in aphasia treatment. In R. Chapey (ed.), *Language intervention strategies in adult aphasia*. Baltimore: Williams & Wilkins.

DEAL, J.L. and FLORANCE, C.L. 1978: Modification of the eight-step continuum for treatment of apraxia of speech in adults. *JSHD* **43**, 89–95.

DE RENZI, E. and FAGLIONI, D. 1978: Normative data and screening power of a shortened version of the Token Test. *Cortex* **14**, 41–9.

DE RENZI, E. and FERRARI, C. 1978: The Reporter's Test: a sensitive test to detect expressive disturbance in aphasics. *Cortex* **14**, 279–93.

DE RENZI, E. and VIGNOLO, L. 1962: The Token Test: a sensitive test to detect receptive disturbances in aphasic. *Brain* **85**, 665–78.

DE SAUSSURE, F. 1916: Cours de linguistique générale. Paris: Payot. (English translation; Course in general linguistics, 1966, New York: McGraw-Hill.)

DIMOND, S.J. 1972: *The double brain*. London: Churchill-Livingstone.

—— 1979: Symmetry and asymmetry in the vertebrate brain. In D.A. Oakley and H.C. Plotkin (eds.), *Brain, behaviour and evolution*. London: Methuen.

DIMOND, S.J. and BEAUMONT, J.G. (eds.), 1974: *Hemispheric function in the human brain*. London: Elek Science.
DUBOIS, J., IRIGARAY, L., MARCIE, P. and HÉCAEN, H. 1967: Pathologie du language. *Languages* **5**, 1–127.
DUFFY, R.J. and BUCK, R.W. 1979: A study of the relationship between propositional (pantomime) and subpropositional (facial expression) extraverbal behaviours in aphasics. *Folia Phoniat.* **31**, 129–36.
EAGLESON, H., VAUGHN, G. and KNUDSON, A. 1970: Hand signals for dysphasics. *Archives of Physical Medicine and Rehabilitation* **51**, 111–13.
EATON GRIFFITH, V. 1975: Volunteer scheme for dysphasia and allied problems in stroke patients. *British Medical Journal* **3**, 633–5.
EGGERT, G.H. 1981: A retrospective view of Wernicke's aphasia. *Aphasia-Apraxia-Agnosia* **2**, 3, 20–32.
EISENSON, J. 1954: *Examining for aphasia*. New York: The Psychological Corporation.
ENDERBY, P. and DAVID, R.M. 1976: Proposed evaluation of speech therapy for acquired aphasia. *BJDC* **11**, 144–8.
ENDERBY, P. and HAMILTON, G. 1979: 'Splink'. A new communication aid for the speech handicapped and deaf. *Paper presented to the Annual Convention of the National Rehabilitation Association of America, 18 September, 1979*.
—— 1981: Clinical trials for communication aids? A study provoked by the clinical trials of SPLINK. *Int. J. Rehab. Research* **4**, 181–95.
FARMER, A. and O'CONNELL, P.F. 1979: Neuropsychological processes in adult aphasia: rationale for treatment. *BJDC* **14**, 39–49.
FAWCUS, M. 1979: Group therapy for the dysphasic patient. *Sprache-Stimme-Gehör* **3**, 12–17.
FILLMORE, C.J. 1968: The case for case. In E. Bach and R.T. Harms (eds.), *Universals in linguistic theory*. New York: Holt, Rinehart & Winston.
FLOWERS, C.R., BEUKELMAN, D.R., BOTTORF, L.E. and KELLEY, R.A. 1979: Family members' predictions of asphasic test performance. *Asphasia-Apraxia-Agnosia* **1**, 18–26.
GARDNER, H. 1976: *The shattered mind*. New York: Vintage Books.
GARDNER, H., ZURIF, E.B., BERRY, T. and BAKER, E. 1976: Visual communication in aphasia. *Neuropsychologia* **11**, 95–103.
GARDENER, R.A. and GARDENER, B.T. 1969: Teaching sign-language to a chimpanzee. *Science* **165**, 664–72.
GAINOTTI, G. 1972: Emotional behavior and hemispheric side of the lesion. *Cortex* **8**, 41–55.
GAZZANIGA, M.S. 1970: *The bisected brain*. New York: Appleton-Century-Crofts.
—— 1975: Brain mechanisms and behaviour. In M.S. Gazzaniga and C. Blakemore (eds.), *Handbook of Psychobiology*. New York: Academic Press.
—— 1977: Consistency and diversity in brain organization. *Annals of the New York Academy of Sciences* **299**, 415–23.
GAZZANIGA, M.S. and LeDOUX, J.E. 1978: *The integrated mind*. New York: Plenum Press.

GAZZANIGA, M.S., LeDOUX, J.E. and WILSON, D.H. 1977: Language, praxis and the right hemisphere: clues to some mechanisms of consciousness. *Neurology* **27**, 1144–7.

GAZZANIGA, M.S., VOLPE, B.T., SMYLIE, C.S. WILSON, D.H. and LeDOUX, J.E. 1979: Plasticity in speech organization following commissurotomy. *Brain* **102**, 805–15.

GESCHWIND, N. 1965: Disconnection syndromes in animals and man. *Brain* **88**, 237–94.

—— 1969: Problems in the anatomical understanding of aphasia. In A.L. Benton (ed.), *Contributions to clinical neurology*. Chicago: Aldine.

—— 1970: The organization of language in the brain. *Science* **170**, 940–4.

—— 1979: Some comments on the neurology of language. In D. Caplan (ed.), *Biological studies of mental processes*. Cambridge, Mass: MIT Press.

GLASS, A.V., GAZZANIGA, M.S. and PREMACK, D. 1973: Artificial language training in global aphasics. *Neuropsychologia* **11**, 95–103.

GLONING, K., TRAPPL, R., HEISS, W.D. and QUATEMBER, R. 1976: Prognosis and speech therapy in aphasia. In Y. Lebrun and R. Hoops (eds.), *Recovery in aphasics*. Amsterdam: Swets & Zeitlinger.

GODFREY, C.M. and DOUGLASS, E. 1959: The recovery process in aphasia. *Canadian Medical Association Journal* **80**, 618–24.

GOLDEN C.J. 1978: *Diagnosis and rehabilitation in clinical neuropsychology*. Springfield, Ill.: Charles C. Thomas.

GOLDSTEIN, H. and CAMERON, H. 1952: New method of communication for the aphasic patient. *Arizona Medicine* **8**, 17–21.

GOODGLASS, H. 1968: Studies on the grammar of aphasics. In S. Rosenberg and J.H. Koplin (eds.), *Developments in applied psycholinguistic research*. New York: Macmillan.

GOODGLASS, H. and BAKER, E. 1976: Semantic field, naming and auditory comprehension in aphasia. *Brain and Language* **3**, 359–74.

GOODGLASS, H., BLUMSTEIN, S.E., GLEASON, J.B., HYDE, M.R., GREEN, E. and STATLENDER, S. 1979: The effect of syntactic encoding on sentence comprehension in aphasia. *Brain and Language* **7**, 201–9.

GOODGLASS, H., GLEASON, J.B., BERNHOLTZ, N.A. and HYDE, M.R. 1972: Some linguistic structures in the speech of a Broca's aphasic. *Cortex* **8**, 191–212.

GOODGLASS, H. and KAPLAN, E. 1963: Disturbance of gesture and pantomime in aphasia. *Brain* **86**, 703–20.

—— 1972: *The assessment of aphasia and related disorders*. Philadelphia: Lea & Febiger.

GOODKIN, R. 1969: Changes in word production, sentence production and relevance in an aphasic through verbal conditioning. *Behaviour Research and Therapy* **7**, 93–9.

GREENBERG, F.R. 1966: Functional communication ability and responses to a structured language test in dysphasic adults. (abstract) *Archives of Physical Medicine and Rehabilitation* **47**, 54.

GREENBLATT, S. 1976: Subangular alexia without agraphia or hemianopsia. *Brain and Language* **3**, 229–45.

GREWEL, F. 1951: Aphasia and linguistics. *Folia Phoniat.* **2**, 100–11.
—— 1963: Prolegomena to patholinguistics. In L. Halpern (ed.), *Problems of dynamic neurology*. Jerusalem: Post Press.
GRUNWELL, P. and DAVIES, C. 1975: A new approach to the treatment of severe dysphasia—a case study. *BJDC* **10**, 142–9.
HAGEN, C. 1973: Communicative abilities in hemiplegia: effect of speech therapy. *Archives of Physical Medicine and Rehabilitation* **54**, 454–65.
HARGIE, O., SAUNDERS, C. and DICKSON, D. 1981: *Social skills in interpersonal communication*. London: Croom Helm.
HARRIS, Z.S. 1951: *Structural linguistics*. Chicago: University of Chicago Press.
HATFIELD, F.M. 1972: Looking for help from linguistics. *BJDC* **7**, 64–81.
—— 1979: Aphasiebehandlung: Methoden und Ansichten. In G. Peuser (ed.), *Studien zur Sprachtherapie* Munich: Wilhelm Fink Verlag.
—— 1980: Verband zwischen schriftlicher und mündlicher Leistung bei einer Erzählaufgabe in zwei Fällen von Aphasie. Paper presented to Meeting of Arbeitsgemeinschaft für Aphasieforschung und-behandlung, 7–8 Nov. 1980 in Maastricht.
HATFIELD, F.M. and ELVIN, M.D. 1978: Die Behandlung des Agrammatismus bei Aphasikern. *Stimme-Sprache-Gehör* **4**, 145–51.
HATFIELD, F.M., HOWARD, D., BARBER, J., JONES, C. and MORTON, J. 1977: Object naming in aphasics—the lack of effect of context or realism. *Neuropsychologia* **15**, 717–27.
HATFIELD, F.M. and PATTERSON, K.E. In Press: Phonological spelling. *Q.J. Exp. Psych.*
HATFIELD, F.M. and WALTON, K. 1975: Phonological patterns in a case of aphasia. *Language and Speech* **18**, 341–57.
HATFIELD, F.M. and WEDDELL, R. 1976: Re-training in writing in severe aphasia. In Y. Lebrun and R. Hoops (eds.). *Recovery in aphasics*. Amsterdam: Swets & Zeitlinger.
HAVIGHURST R.J. 1968: Personality and patterns of ageing. In S.M. Chown (ed.), *Human ageing*. Harmondsworth: Penguin, 1972.
HEAD, H. 1926: *Aphasia and kindred disorders of speech*. Cambridge: CUP.
HEARD, D.H. 1978: From object relations to attachment theory: a basis for family therapy. *Brit. J. Med. Psych.* **51**, 67–76.
HÉCAEN, H. and KREMIN, H. 1976: Neurolonguistic research on reading disorders resulting from left-hemisphere lesions: aphasic and 'pure' alexias. In H. Whitaker and H.A. Whitaker (eds.), *Studies in neurolinguistics. Vol. II*. New York: Academic Press.
HEGDE, M.N., NOLL, M.J. and PECORA, R. 1979: A study of some factors affecting generalization of language training. *JSHD.* **44**, 301–20.
HELM, N. 1979: *A syntax retrieval programme for agrammatic aphasia*. Proceedings of the 8th National Conference of the College of Speech Therapists, Warwick.
HELMICK, J.W. and MARQUARDT, T.P. 1979: Communication of information to the aphasic patient and family. *Allied Health and Behavioral Sciences* **2**, 273–86.

HELMICK, J.W., WATAMORI, T.S. and PALMER, J.M. 1976: Spouses' understanding of the communication disabilities of aphasic patients. *JSHD* **41**, 238–43.
—— 1977: Reply to Holland's comment on 'Spouses' understanding of the communication disabilities of aphasic patients'. *JSHD* **42**, 308–10.
HERON, J. 1977: *Catharsis in human development*. London: Brit. Postgrad. Medical Federation, Univ. London.
HERSEN, M. and BARLOW, D.H. 1976: *Single case experimental designs*. Oxford: Pergamon Press.
HINDE, R.A. (ed.), 1972: *Nonverbal communication* New York: Cambridge University Press.
HJELMSLEV, L. 1953: *Prolegomena to a theory of language*. (Translated from Danish, 1943, by F.J. Whitfield.) Bloomington: Indiana University Press.
HODGINS, E. 1968: *Episode-report on the accident inside my skull*. New York: Atheneum.
HOLLAND, A. 1970: Case studies in aphasia rehabilitation using programmed instruction. *JSHD* **35**, 377–90.
HOLLAND, A.L. 1975: The effectiveness of treatment in aphasia. In R.M. Brookshire (ed.), *Clinical aphasiology conference proceedings 1975*. Minneapolis: BRK Publishers.
—— 1977: Comment on 'Spouses' understanding of the communication disabilities of aphasic patients'. *JSHD* **42**, 307–8.
HOLLAND, A.L. and HARRIS, A.B. 1968: Aphasia rehabilitation using programmed instruction. In H. Sloane and B.D. MacAulay (eds.), *Operant procedures in remedial speech and language training*. Boston: Houghton Mifflin.
HOPKINS, A. 1975: The need for speech therapy for dysphasia following stroke. *Health Trends* **7**, 58–60.
HUSKINS, S.M. 1979: *Differential diagnosis between asphasic phonological impairment and articulatory dyspraxia: implications for planning treatment*. Proceedings of the 8th National Conference of the College of Speech Therapists, Warwick.
JACKSON, H. 1874: On the nature of the duality of the brain. *Brain* **38**, 80–6.
JAKOBSON, R. 1956: Two aspects of language and two types of aphasic disturbances. In R. Jacobson and M. Halle (eds.), *Fundamentals of language*. The Hague: Mouton.
—— 1964: Towards a linguistic typology of aphasic impairments. In A.V.S. De Reuck and M. O'Connor (eds.), *Disorders of language*. London: Churchill.
—— 1968: *Child language, aphasia and phonological universals*. Janua Linguarum Series Minor 72. The Hague: Mouton.
JAKOBSON, R. and HALLE, M. 1956: *Fundamentals of language*. The Hague: Mouton.
JENKINS, J.J., JIMÉNEZ-PABÓN, E., SHAW, R. and WILLIAMS, J. 1975: *Schuell's aphasia in adults diagnosis, prognosis and treatment*, (2nd edn). New York: Harper & Row.
JOHNS, D.F. and LaPOINTE, L.L. 1976: Neurogenic disorders of output processing: apraxia of speech. In H. Whitaker and H.A. Whitaker (eds.), *Studies in neurolinguistics*, vol. 1. New York: Academic Press.

JOHNSON, J.P., SOMMERS, R.K. and WEIDNER, W.E. 1977: Dichotic ear preference in asphasia. *JSHR* **20**, 116–29.
KEAN, M-L, 1977: The linguistic interpretation of aphasic syndromes: agrammatism in Broca's aphasia, an example. *Cognition 5*, 9–46.
—— 1978: The linguistic interpretation of the aphasic syndromes. In E. Walker (ed.), *Explorations in the biology of language*. Montgomery, Vt: Bradford Books.
KEENAN, J.S. 1979: Selecting therapy goals for aphasic patients. *Aphasia-Apraxia-Agnosia* **1**, 32–8.
KELLY, G.A. 1955: *The psychology of personal constructs*. New York: Norton.
KENIN, M. and SWISHER, L. 1972: A study of pattern of recovery in aphasia. *Cortex* **8**, 56–68.
KERSHNER, J., THOMAE, R. and CALLAWAY, R. 1977: Nonverbal fixation control in young children induces a left-field advantage in digit recall. *Neuropsychologia* **15**, 569–76.
KERTESZ, A. and MCCABE, P. 1977: Recovery patterns and prognosis in aphasia. *Brain* **100**, 1–18.
KERTESZ, A. and POOLE, E. 1974: The Aphasia Quotient: the taxonomic approach to measurement of aphasic disability. *Canadian Journal of Neurological Sciences* **1**, 7–16.
KIMURA, D. 1973: The asymmetry of the human brain. *Scientific American* **228**, 70–80.
KIMURA, D. and ARCHIBALD, Y. 1974: Motor functions of the left hemisphere. *Brain* **97**, 337–50.
KINSBOURNE, M. 1971: The minor cerebral hemisphere as a source of aphasic speech. *Arch. Neurol.* **25**, 302–6.
KINSELLA, G. and DUFFY, F.D. 1978: The spouse of the asphasic patient. In Y. Lebrun and R. Hoops (eds.) *The management of aphasia*. Amsterdam: Swets & Zeitlinger.
—— 1979: Psychosocial readjustment in the spouses of aphasic patients. *Scand. J. Rehab. Medicine* **11**, 129–32.
—— 1980: Attitudes towards disability expressed by spouses of stroke patients. *Scand. J. Rehab. Medicine* **12**, 73–6.
KOPP, S. 1972: *If you meet the Buddha on the road, kill him!* London: Sheldon Press.
KOTTEN, A. 1977: *Differences in identification of spatial and temporal prepositions*. Unpublished paper presented to the AAFB Conference, Bonn. (In German.)
—— 1979: *Umweg-und Stützfunktion des Schreibens in der Therapie*. Paper presented to Meeting of AAFB, Nov., Aachen.
KRAETSCHMER, K. 1981: A re-examination of Broca's contribution to neurological research. *Aphasia-Apraxia-Agnosia* **2**, 7–19.
KREMIN, H. 1980: *Lexikalische Agraphie: eine selektive Störung der Orthographie?* Paper presented to Meeting of AAFB, 7–8 Nov., Maastricht.
KUBLER-ROSS, E. 1970: *On death and dying*. London: Tavistock.

KUČERA, H. and FRANCIS, W.N. 1967: *Computational analysis of present-day American English*. Providence, RI: Brown University Press.

LaPOINTE, L.L. 1977: Base 10 programmed stimulation: test specification, scoring and plotting performance in aphasia therapy. *JSHD* **42**, 90–105.

—— 1978: Aphasia therapy: some principles and strategies for treatment, in D.F. Johns (ed.), *Clinical management of neurologic communicative disorders*. Boston: Little, Brown & Co.

LARSEN, B., SKINHØJ, E. and LASSEN, N. 1978: Variations in regional cortical blood flow in the right and left hemispheres during automatic speech. *Brain* **101**, 193–209.

LASHLEY, K. 1929: *Brain mechanisms and intelligence*. Chicago: UCP.

LASSEN, N.A., INGVAR, D.H. and SKINHØJ, E. 1978: Brain function and blood flow. *Scientific American* **239**, 50–9.

LAURENCE, S. and STEIN, D.G. 1978: Recovery after brain damage and the concept of localization of function. In S. Finger (ed.), *Recovery from brain damage*. New York: Plenum Press.

LENNEBERG, E.H. 1974: Language and brain: developmental aspects. *Neurosciences Research Programme Bulletin* **12**, 511–656.

LESSER, R. 1974: Verbal comprehension in aphasia: an English version of three Italian tests. *Cortex* **10**, 247–63.

—— 1978: *Linguistic investigations of aphasia*. London: Edward Arnold.

LeVERE, T.E. 1975: Neural stability, sparing, and behavioural recovery following brain damage. *Psychological Review* **82**, 344–58.

—— 1980: Recovery of function after brain damage: a theory of the behavioural deficit. *Physiological Psychology* **8**, 297–308.

LEVITA, E. 1978: Effects of speech therapy on aphasics' responses to Functional Communication Profile. *Perceptual Motor Skills* **47**, 151–4.

LEVY, J. 1969: Possible basis for the evolution of lateral specialization of the human brain. *Nature* **224**, 614–15.

LEZAK, M. 1976: *Neuropsychological assessment*. New York: Oxford University Press.

LIBERMAN, R.P. and TEIGEN J. 1979: Behavioral group therapy. In P.O. Sjödén, S. Bates and W.S. Dockens (eds.), *Trends in behavior therapy*. New York: Academic Press.

LOMAS, J. and KERTESZ. A. 1978: Patterns of spontaneous recovery in aphasic groups: a study of adult stroke patients. *Brain and Language* **5**, 388–401.

LORBER, J. 1980: *Is your brain really necessary?* Paper presented to the British Paediatric Association Annual Conference, York, England.

LURIA, A.R. 1963: *Restoration of brain function after brain injury*. New York: Macmillan.

—— 1966: *Higher cortical functions in man*. London: Tavistock.

—— 1970: *traumatic aphasia*. The Hague: Mouton.

—— 1973: *The working brain*. Harmondsworth: Penguin.

LURIA, A.R., NAYDIN, V.L., TSVETKOVA, L.S. and VINANKAYA, E.N. 1969: Restoration of higher cortical function following local brain damage. In R.J. Vinken and

G.W. Bruyn (eds.), *Handbook of clinical neurology*, vol. 3. Amsterdam: North Holland.

LYONS, J. 1963: *Structural semantics*. Oxford: Blackwell.

MacMAHON, M.K.C. 1972: Modern linguistics and aphasia. *BJDC* **7**, 54–63.

MALONE, R., PTACEK, P. and MALONE, M. 1970: Attitudes expressed by families of aphasics. *BJDC* **5**, 174–9.

MARKS, M., TAYLOR, H. and RUSK, H. 1957: Rehabilitation of the aphasic patient: a survey of three years experience in a rehabilitation setting. *Neurology* **7**, 837–43.

MARSHALL, J.C. 1973: Some problems and paradoxes associated with recent accounts of hemispheric specialization. *Neuropsychologia* **11**, 463–70.

MARSHALL, J.C. and NEWCOMBE, F. 1966: Syntactic and semantic errors in paralexia. *Neuropsychologia* **4**, 169–76.

—— 1973: Patterns of paralexia: a psycholinguistic approach. *Journal of Psycholinguistic Research* **2**, 175–200.

—— 1977: Variability and constraint in acquired dyslexia. In H. Whitaker and H.A. Whitaker (eds.), *Studies in neurolinguistics, vol. III*. New York: Academic Press.

MEIKLE, M., WECHSLER, E., TUPPER, A., BENNENSON, M., BUTLER, J., MULHALL, D. and STERN, G. 1979: Comparative trial of volunteer and professional treatments of dysphasia after stroke. *British Medical Journal* **2**, 87–9.

MEYERSON, R. and GOODGLASS, H. 1972: Transformational grammars of aphasic patients. *Language and Speech* **15**, 40–50.

MILLER, G.A., GALANTER, E. and PRIBRAM, K.H. 1960: *Plans and the Structure of Behaviour*. London: Holt, Rinehart & Winston.

MILLS, L. and ROLLMAN, G.B. 1979: Left hemisphere selectivity for processing duration in normal subjects. *Brain and Language* **7**, 320–35.

—— 1980: Hemispheric asymmetry for auditory perception of temporal order. *Neuropsychologia* **18**, 41–7.

MILNER, B. 1974: Hemispheric specialization: scope and limits. In F.O. Schmitt and F.G. Worden (eds.), *The neurosciences: third study programme*. Cambridge, Mass: MIT Press.

MOLLON, P. 1979: Transforming anxiety. *New Forum* **5**, 59–61.

MOORE, W.H. and WEIDNER, W. 1974: Bilateral tachistoscopic word perception in aphasic and normal subjects. *Perceptual and Motor Skills* **39**, 1003–11.

—— 1975: Dichotic word perception of aphasic and normal subjects. *Perceptual and Motor Skills* **40**, 379–86.

MORTON, J. 1980: The logogen model and orthographic structure. In U. Frith (ed.), *Cognitive processes in spelling*. London: Academic Press.

MORTON, J. and PATTERSON, K. 1980a: 'Little Words—No!' In M. Coltheart, K. Patterson and J.C. Marshall (eds.), *Deep dyslexia*. London: Routledge & Kegan Paul.

—— 1980b: A new attempt at an interpretation, or, an attempt at a new interpretation. In M. Coltheart, K. Patterson and J.C. Marshall (eds.), *Deep dyslexia*. London: Routledge & Kegan Paul.

MULHALL, D.J. 1978: Dysphasic stroke patients and the influence of their relatives. *BJDC* **13**, 127–34.

MÜLLER, D.J., MUNRO, S. and CODE, C. 1981: *Language assessment for remediation*. London: Croom Helm.

MURRELL, G.A. and MORTON, J. 1974: Word recognition and morphemic structure. *J. Exp. Psych.* **102**, 963–8.

NAESER, M.A. 1975: A structured approach teaching aphasics basic sentence types. *BJDC* **10**, 70–7.

NEBES, R.D. 1973: Perception of dot patterns by the disconnected right and left hemisphere in man. *Neuropsychologia* **11**, 285–90.

NEWELL, A., SHAW, J. and SIMON, H. 1961: Computer simulation of human thinking. *Science* **134**, 2011–17.

NEWSON, J. and NEWSON, E. 1976: *Seven years old in the home environment*. London: Allen & Unwin.

NIELSEN, J.M. 1946: *Agnosia, apraxia, aphasia: their value in cerebral localization*. New York: Hoeber.

OJEMANN, G.A. 1975: Language and the thalamus; object naming and recall during and after thalamic stimulation. *Brain and Language* **2**, 101–20.

OJEMANN, G.A. and WHITAKER, H.A. 1978a: Language localization and variability. *Brain and Language* **6**, 239–60.

—— 1978b: The bilingual brain. *Archives of Neurology* **35**, 409–12.

OLDFIELD, R.G. 1971: The assessment and analysis of handedness: The Edinburgh Inventory. *Neuropsychologia* **9**, 97–113.

OSCAR-BERMAN, M., REHBEIN, L., PORFERT, A and GOODGLASS, H. 1978: Dichhaptic hand-order effects with verbal and nonverbal tactile stimulation. *Brain and Language* **6**, 323–33.

OSTREICHER, H.V. 1980: The use of simultaneous gestural-verbal techniques with aphasic and apraxic adults. *Aphasia-Apraxia-Agnosia* **2**, 31–44.

PARISI, D. and PIZZAMIGLIO, L. 1970: Syntactic comprehension in aphasia. *Cortex* **6**, 204–15.

PARKES, C.M. 1975: *Bereavement: studies of grief in adult life*. Harmondsworth: Penguin.

PATTERSON, K. 1978: Phonemic dyslexia: errors of meaning and the meaning of errors. *Q. J. of Exp. Psych.* **30**, 587–601.

—— 1979: What is right with deep dyslexic patients? *Brain and Language* **8**, 111–29.

—— 1981: Neuropsychological approaches to the study of reading. *B. J. Psych.* **72**, 151–74.

PATTERSON, K, and MARCEL, A.J. 1977: Aphasia, dyslexia and the phonological coding of written words. *Q. J. Exp. Psych.* **29**, 307–18.

PEASE MYERS, D. and GOODGLASS, H. 1978: The effects of cueing on picture naming in aphasia. *Cortex* **14**, 178–89.

PENFIELD, W. and ROBERTS, L. 1959: *Speech and brain mechanisms*. Princeton, N.J: Princeton University Press.

PETTIT, J.M. and NOLL, J.D. 1979: Cerebral dominance in aphasia recovery. *Brain and Language* **7**, 191–200.
POPPER, K.R. and ECCLES, J.C. 1977: *The self and its brain*. New York: Springer International.
PORCH, B.E. 1967: *Porch index of communicative ability; volume 1: Theory and development*. Palo Alto: Consulting Psychologists' Press.
—— 1971: *Porch index of communicative ability; volume 2: Administration, scoring and interpretation*. Palo Alto: Consulting Psychologists' Press.
POWELL, G.E. 1981: *Brain function therapy*. Farnham: Teakfield.
POWELL, G., CLARK, E. and BAILEY, S. 1979: Categories of aphasia: a cluster analysis of Schuell test profiles. *BJDC* **14**, 111–22.
PREMACK, D. 1971: Language in chimpanzee? *Science* **172**, 808–22.
PRINS, R.S., SNOW, C.E. and WAGENAAR, E. 1978: Recovery from aphasia: spontaneous speech versus language comprehension. *Brain and Language* **6**, 192–211.
PRINZ, P.M. 1980: A note on requesting strategies in adult aphasics. *J. Com. Dis.* **13**, 65–73.
QUIRK, R. and GREENBAUM, S. 1973: *A university grammar of English*. London: Longman.
RAVEN, J.C. 1938a: *Coloured progressive matrices*. London: H.K. Lewis.
—— 1938b: *Standard progressive matrices*. London: H.K. Lewis.
REINVANG, I. 1969: Functional language in aphasia. *Scand. J. Rehab. Medicine* **1**, 112–16.
RICHARDSON, J.T.E. 1976a: Effects of stimulus attributes on latency of word recognition. *B.J. Psych.* **67**, 315–25.
—— 1976b: The effect of word imageability in acquired dyslexia. *Neuropsychologia* **13**, 281–8.
ROCHFORD, G. and WILLIAMS, M. 1962: Studies in the development and breakdown of the use of names, i: The relationship between nominal dysphasia and the acquisition of vocabulary in childhood. ii: Experimental production of naming disorders in normal people. *J. Neurol., Neurosurg. Psychiat.* **25**, 222–33.
—— 1963: iii: Recovery from nominal dysphasia. *J. Neurol. Neurosurg. and Psychiat.* **26**, 377–81.
—— 1965: iv: The effects of word frequency. *J. Neurol. Neurosurg. Psychiat.* **28**, 407–13.
ROCKEY, D. 1973: *Phonetic lexicon*. London: Heyden & Son.
ROGERS, C.R. 1951: *Client-centred therapy*. London: Constable.
ROSENBEK, J.C., LEMME, M.L., AHEARN, M.B., HARRIS, E.H. and WERTZ, R.T. 1973: A treatment for apraxia of speech in adults. *JSHD.* **38**, 462–72.
ROSNER, B.S. 1974: Recovery of function and localization of function in historical perspective. In D.G. Stein, J.J. Rosen and N. Butters (eds.), *Plasticity and recovery of function in the CNS*. New York: Academic Press.
ROSS, A.J. 1979: A Study of the application of Blissymbolics as a means of communication for a young brain-damaged adult. *BJDC* **14**, 103–9.

ROSS, E.D. and MESULAM, M-M. 1979: Dominant language functions of the right hemisphere? Prosody and emotional gesturing. *Arch. Neurol.* **36**, 144–8.

ROZIN, P., PORITSKY, S. and SOTSKY, R. 1971: The use of Chinese ideographs in training dyslexic children. *Science* **3977**, 1264–7.

SAFFRAN, E.M. 1982: Neuropsychological approaches to the study of language. *B. J. Psych.*, **73**, 317–37.

SARNO, M.T. 1969: *The functional communication profile: manual of directions*. Rehabilitation Monograph 42. New York: Institute of Rehabilitation Medicine.

—— 1976: The status of research in recovery from aphasia. In Y. Lebrun, and R. Hoops (eds.), *Recovery in Aphasics*. Amsterdam: Swets & Zeitlinger.

—— 1980a: Review of research in aphasia: recovery and rehabilitation. In M.T. Sarno and O. Höök (eds.), *Aphasia: assessment and treatment*. New York: Masson.

—— 1980b: Aphasia rehabilitation. In M.T. Sarno and O. Höök (eds.), *Aphasia: assessment and treatment*. New York: Masson.

SARNO, M.T. and LEVITA, E. 1979: Recovery in treated aphasia in the first year post-stroke. *Stroke* **10**, 663–70.

SARNO, M.T., SILVERMAN, M.G. and SANDS, F.S. 1970: Speech therapy and language recovery in severe aphasia. *JSHR* **13**, 607–23.

SAYA, M. 1979: Blissymbolics: an alternative system of communication for the non-verbal aphasic patient. Paper presented at Canadian Speech and Hearing Association Conference.

SCHLANGER, P. 1976: Training the adult aphasic to pantomime. Paper presented at 51st Annual Meeting of the America Speech and Hearing Association, Houston.

SCHLANGER, P. and FREIMANN, R. 1979: Pantomime therapy with aphasics. *Aphasia-Apraxia-Agnosia* **1**, 34–9.

SCHNITZER, M.L. 1978: Toward a neurolinguistic theory of language. *Brain and Language* **6**, 342–61.

SCHUELL, H. 1965: *The Minnesota test for the differential diagnosis of aphasia*. Minneapolis: Univ. Minnesota Press.

SCHUELL, H. and BREWER, R.S. 1969: A psycholinguistic approach to study of the language deficit in aphasia. *JSHR* **12**, 794–806.

SCHUELL, H., JENKINS, J. and JIMÉNEZ-PABON, E. 1964: *Aphasia in adults*. New York: Harper & Row.

SEARLEMAN, A. 1977: A review of right-hemisphere linguistic capabilities. *Psychological Bulletin* **84**, 503–28.

SELIGMAN, M.E.P. 1975: *Helplessness: on depression, development and death*. San Francisco: Freeman.

SERON, X., DELOCHE, G., BASTARD, V., CHASSIN, G. and HERMAND, N. 1979: Word-finding difficulties in learning transfer in aphasic patients. *Cortex* **15**, 149–55.

SERON, X., DELOCHE, G., MOULARD, G. and ROUSSELE, M. 1980: A computer-based therapy for the treatment of aphasic subjects with writing disorders. *JSHD* **45**, 45–58.

SHAI, A., GOODGLASS, H. and BARTON, M. 1972: Recognition of tachistoscopically presented verbal and nonverbal material after unilateral cerebral damage. *Neuropsychologia* **10**, 185–91.
SILVERMAN, F.H. 1980: *Communication for the speechless*. Englewood Cliffs, NJ: Prentice Hall, Inc.
SKELLY, M., SCHINSKY, L., SMITH, R.W. and FUST, R.S. 1974: American Indian Sign Language (Amerind) as a facilitator for the oral-verbal apraxic. *JSHD* **39**, 445–56.
SKINHØJ, E. and LARSEN, B. 1980: The pattern of cortical activation during speech and listening in normal and different types of aphasic patients as revealed by regional cerebral blood flow (CBF). In M.T. Sarno and C. Hook (eds.), *Aphasia: assessment and treatment*. New York: Masson.
SMAIL, D.J. 1978: *Psychotherapy: A personal approach*. London: Dent.
SMITH, A. 1966: Speech and other functions after left (dominant) hemispherectomy. *J. Neurol., Neurosurg. Psychiat.* **29**, 467–71.
—— 1972: *Diagnosis, intelligence and rehabilitation of chronic aphasics*. Ann Arbor: University of Michigan Department of Physical Medicine and Rehabilitation.
SNODGRASS, J.G. and VANDERVART, M. 1980: A standardized set of 260 pictures: norms for name agreement, image agreement, familiarity and visual complexity. *Journal of Experimental Psychology: Human Learning and Memory* **6**, 174–215.
SOH, K., LARSEN, B., SKINHØJ, E. and LASSEN, N.A. 1978: Regional cerebral blood flow in aphasia. *Arch. Neurol.* **35**, 625–32.
SPARKS, R.W. and HOLLAND, A.L. 1976: Method: melodic intonation therapy for aphasia. *JSHD* **41**, 287–97.
SPERRY, R.W. 1965: Mind, brain and humanist values. In J.R. Platt (ed.), *New views on the nature of man*. Chicago: UCP.
SPERRY, R.W. 1966: Brain bisection and mechanisms of consciousness. In J.C. Eccles (ed.), *Brain and conscious experience*. New York: Springer-Verlag.
—— 1970: Perception in the absence of the neocortical commissures. *Perception and its disorders, Research Publication 48*. The Association for Research in Mental and Nervous Disease.
—— 1979: Consciousness, freewill and personal identity. In D.A. Oakley and H.C. Plotkin (eds.), *Brain, behaviour and evolution*. London: Methuen.
SPINNLER, H. and VIGNOLO, L. 1966: Impaired recognition of meaningful sounds in aphasia. *Cortex* **2**, 337–48.
SPOEHR, K.T. 1978: Phonological encoding in visual word recognition. *JVLVB* **17**, 127–41.
SPREEN, O. and BENTON, A.L. 1969: *Neurosensory center comprehensive examination for aphasia: manual of directions*. University of Victoria, Neuropsychology Laboratory.
STEIN, D.G., ROSEN, J.J. and BUTTERS, N. 1974: *Plasticity and recovery of function in the CNS*. New York: Academic Press.
STORR, A. 1979: *The art of psychotherapy*. London: Heinemann.

TALLAL, P. and NEWCOMBE, F. 1978: Impairment of auditory perception and language comprehension in dysphasia. *Brain and Language* **5**, 13–24.

TANNER, D.C. 1980: Loss and grief. Implications for the speech-language pathologist and audiologist. *Asha* **22**, 916–28.

TAYLOR, M.L. 1964: Language therapy. In H.G. Burr (ed.), *The aphasic adult: evaluation and rehabilitation*. Charlottesville Va: Wayside Press.

—— 1965: A measurement of functional communication in aphasia. *Archives of Physical Medicine and Rehabilitation* **46**, 101–7.

THOMPSON, J. 1978: Cognitive effects of cortical lesions. In B. Foss (ed.), *Psychology survey* no. 1. London: Allen & Unwin.

TRIM, J. 1963: Linguistics and speech pathology. In S.E. Mason (ed.), *Signs, signals and symbols*. London: Methuen.

—— 1965: *English pronunciation illustrated*. Cambridge: Cambridge University Press.

TROWER, P., BRYANT, B. and ARGYLE, M. 1978: *Social skills and mental health*. London: Methuen.

TSVETKOVA, L.S. 1975: The naming process and its impairment. In E.H. Lenneberg and E. Lenneberg (eds.), *Foundations of language development*, vol. 2. London: Academic Press.

VARNEY, N.R. 1980: Sound recognition in relation to aural language comprehension in aphasic patients. *J. Neurol., Neurosurg., Psychiat.* **43**, 71–5.

VIGNOLO, L.A. 1964: Evolution of aphasia and language rehabilitation: a retrospective exploratory study. *Cortex* **1**, 344–67.

WADA, J.A. and RASMUSSEN, T. 1960: Intracarotid injection of sodium amytal for the lateralization of cerebral speech dominance. Experimental and clinical observations. *J. Neurosurg.* **17**, 266–82.

WALKER, M. 1976: The Makaton vocabulary: a progress report. *Apex* **3**, 27–8.

WALSH, K.W. 1978: *Neuropsychology: a clinical approach*. Edinburgh: Churchill Livingstone.

WARREN, C.E.J. and MORTON, J. 1982: The effects of priming on picture recognition. *B. J. Psych.* **73**, 117–29.

WARRINGTON, E.K. 1975: The selective impairment of semantic memory. *Q. J. Exp. Psych.* **27**, 635–57.

WEIGL, E. 1961: The phenomenon of temporary deblocking in aphasia. *Zeitschrift für Phonetische Sprachwissenschaft und Kommunikationsforschung* **14**, 337–61.

—— 1970: A neuropsychological contribution to the study of semantics. In M. Bierwisch and E.E. Heidolph (eds.), *Progress in linguistics*. The Hague: Mouton.

—— 1972: Zur Schriftsprache und ihrem Erwerb—neuropsychologische und psycholinguistische Betrachtungen. *Probleme. Ergebnisse der Psychologie* **43**, 45–105.

WEIGL, E. and BIERWISCH, M. 1970: Neuropsychology and linguistics: topics of common research. *Foundations of Language* **6**, 1–18.

WEIGL, E. and FRADIS, A. 1977: The transcoding processes in patients with agraphia to dictation. *Brain and Language* **4**, 11–22.
WELFORD, A.T. 1968: *Fundamentals of skill*. London: Methuen.
WERNICKE, C. 1874: Der aphasische Symptomencomplex. Breslau: Cohn & Weigert.
WERTZ, R.T., COLLINS, M.J., WEISS, D., BROOKSHIRE, R.H., FRIDEN, T., KURTZKE, J.F. and PIERCE, J. 1978: *The veterans administration co-operative study on aphasia: A comparison of individual and group treatment*. Presentation to the Academy of Aphasia.
WHITAKER, H.A. and WHITAKER, H. 1979: Lexical, syntactic and semantic aspects of the Token Test: a linguistic taxonomy. In F. Boller and M. Dennis (eds.), *Auditory comprehension: clinical and experimental studies with the Token Test*. London: Academic Press.
WHITEHEAD, S. 1973: A comparison of the efficacy of intensive, group therapy with that of non-intensive, individual speech therapy for adult dysphasics. Unpublished thesis in part fulfilment of the MSc in the Guy's Hospital Medical School, University of London.
WHURR, R. 1974: *An aphasia screening test*. Reading: University of Reading.
WIEGEL-CRUMP, C. 1976: Agrammatism and aphasia. In Y. Lebrun and R. Hoops (eds.), *Recovery in aphasics*. Amsterdam: Swets & Zeitlinger.
WIEGEL-CRUMP, C. and KOENIGSKNECHT, R.A. 1973: Tapping the lexical store of the adult aphasic: Analysis of the improvement made in word retrieval skills. *Cortex* **9**, 410–17.
WINNICOTT, D.W. 1964: *The child, the family, and the outside world*. Harmondsworth: Penguin.
—— 1971: *Playing and reality*. London: Tavistock.
WOODS, B.T. and PÖPPEL, E. 1974: Effect of print size on reading time in a patient with verbal alexia. *Neuropsychologia* **12**, 31–41.
WULF, H.H. 1973: *Aphasia, my world alone*. Detroit: Wayne State Univ. Press.
YULE, W. and HEMSLEY, D. 1977: Single-case method in medical psychology. In S. Rachman (ed.), *Contributions to medical psychology*, vol, 1. Oxford: Pergamon Press.
ZAIDEL, E. 1973: Linguistic competence and related functions in the right hemisphere of man following cerebral commissurotomy and hemispherectomy. PhD thesis, California Institute of Technology, Pasadena, USA.
—— 1974: Language, dichotic listening and the disconnected hemispheres. Paper presented at the Conference on Human Brain Function, University of California, Los Angeles.
—— 1976: Auditory vocabulary of the right hemisphere following brain bisection or hemicortication. *Cortex* **12**, 191–211.
—— 1978: Auditory language comprehension in the right hemisphere following cerebral commissurotomy and hemispherectomy: a comparison with child language and aphasia. In A. Caramazza and E.B Zurif (eds.), *Language*

acquisition and language breakdown. Baltimore: Johns Hopkins University Press.

ZANGWILL, O.L. 1975: The relation of nonverbal cognitive functions to aphasia. In E.H. Lenneberg and E. Lenneberg (eds.), *Foundations of language development*, vol. 2. London: Academic Press.

ZURIF, E.B. and CARAMAZZA, A. 1976: Psycholinguistic structures in aphasia studies in syntax and semantics. In H. and H.A. Whitaker (eds.), *Studies in neurolinguistics*, vol. 1. New York: Academic Press.

Subject Index

Agnosia, 8, 45, 77
   acoustic, 138, 140
   visual, 146
Agnosic alexia, 146
Agrammatism, 4, 159, 166, 169, 198
   therapy for, 69–74
Agraphia (and dysgraphia), 8, 127, 157–69, 190, 192
   deep dysgraphia 158, 161
   diagnostic tests for, 158–63
   information-processing model of, 157
   paragraphia, 161
      semantic, 161
      derivational, 161, 162
   phonological, 158
   surface (lexical or orthographic), 158
   therapy for
      deep dysgraphia, 164–8
      surface dysgraphia, 165–8
Alcoholism, 124
Alexia (and dyslexia), 8, 146–56, 157
   anterior (deep or phonemic), 146, 157, 159, 161
   as disconnection syndrome, 146
   assessment and differential diagnosis of, 147–8
   as visual agnosia, 146
   central (alexia with agraphia), 146
   letter-by-letter reading, 157
   paralexia, 157
   phonological, 157
   prognosis of, 148, 156
   pure (agnosic alexia, alexia without agraphia, posterior, pure word blindness, subcortical alexia, visual alexia), 146
   surface, 157
   the syndrome of, 147
   therapy for, 148–56
      Cloze procedure in 155
      look-cover-write-check procedure in, 154
      split-sentence technique in, 152
      visual and auditory memory in, 154
Alternative communication methods, 4, 7, 130, 131, 170, 170–92, 171–5, 178, 194
Amerind, 130, 132, 133
Aphasia, anatomical explanations for, 76
Aphasia therapist as researcher, 193, 194–202
Aphasia therapy research, 193, 194–202
Aphasia types
   afferent, 128, 131
   anomia, 4, 8, 18, 53, 63, 77, 86, 103
   Broca's, 8, 18, 43, 63, 64, 65, 66, 67
   conduction, 18, 64, 67, 198
   efferent, 128
   global, 4, 22, 43, 115, 158
   sensory, therapy for, 127, 138–45
      acoustic analysis in, 140–3
      associated writing impairment in, 138
      auditory training in, 141–3, 144–5
      phonemic hearing impairment in, 138–40, 156
   transcortical motor, 18
   transcortical sensory, 18
   Wernicke's, 18, 44, 56, 63, 65, 67, 74, 77, 95, 105
   with persisting dysfluency, 128
   with sensorimotor impairment, 128
Aphasia quotient, 18
Apraxia, 6, 8, 10, 121
   buccofacial, 129, 130
   ideomotor, 129, 130, 131, 133
   oral, 130, 131
Apraxia of speech (articulatory apraxia, verbal apraxia), 127, 128–37, 156, 178, 186, 190, 197
   differential diagnosis of, 128
   therapy for, 129–37
Articulation drills, 136
Articulograms (and articulatory diagrams), 131, 132, 133, 140, 141, 142
Artificial languages, 4, 36, 42, 43, 59, 170, 171–5
Assessment, 10, 11–12
   baseline, 10
   criterion-referenced profiles, 12
   in efficacy studies, 18–20, 194, 202
   mental test, 27
   of agraphia, 158–63
   of alexia, 147–8
   ongoing evaluation, 4, 11–12, 41
Asymmetry of function, 29, 30–1, 42
Automatic vs voluntary responses, 41

Base 10 format, 10, 11, 47, 48, 50
Behavioural methodology 4, 38, 10–11 (*see also* systematic behavioural perspective)
   cueing, 10
   fading, 4, 10, 11
   feedback, 117, 118, 128
   knowledge of results, 117–18
   modelling, 10
   programmed instruction, 10, 19, 20, 35
   prompting, 4, 10, 11
   reinforcement, 4, 10, 11, 35, 116–17, 118
   stimulus-response, 10, 41
Behaviourism, 27
Blissymbolics, 43, 130, 170, 177, 178–86, 194
   and group therapy, 180, 182
   and the right hemisphere, 184, 185, 186
Brain damage, general and specific effects of, 28

SUBJECT INDEX

Brain Function Therapy, 38
Broca's aphemia, 128

Canon communicator, 175–7
Collateral sprouting, 33
Communication aids, 170, 175–7, 194
  Canon Communicator, 175–7
  clinical trials for, 187–91
  Language Master, 175–7
  Lightwriter, 175–7
  personal computers, 175, 176–7
  Possum Communicator, 175–6
  Speak and Spell, 175–6
  Splink, 170, 175, 176, 187–92
Compensation, 34
Compensatory strategies, 43
Comprehension deficit, 45, 57, 59
  auditory verbal retention in, 45, 46, 47, 55, 57
  phonemic discrimination in, 45, 46, 47, 138–9
  temporal processing in, 45
Computer-based methods 10 (*see also* personal computers)
Counselling, 107, 137
Cross-modal processing, 29, 46, 53
Crossover-treatment design in aphasia therapy, 200

Deblocking, 5, 41, 67, 85, 163
Dementia, 124
Depression, 94, 122
Diaschisis, 32
Dichotic listening, 30, 36, 37, 43, 44, 45–7, 55, 56, 57, 59
Disconnection model and syndromes, 29, 146
Dominance shift (*see* lateral shift)
Dualism, 40–1
Dysarthria, 128, 190
Dysgraphia (*see* agraphia)
Dyslexia (*see* alexia)
Dysphasia (*see* aphasia)
Dyspraxia (*see* apraxia)

Efficacy of aphasia therapy, 12, 14–24, 74, 193, 194–202
Efficacy research, 14–24, 104 193, 194–202
  crossover-treatment design for, 200
  intensive treatment in, 22–3, 63
  large-scale studies of, 14–24, 193
  long-term treatment in, 22–3
  multicentre trials in, 18, 21
  permanence of effects of therapy, 200–1
  single-case study approach to, 193, 194–202
  subject selection in, 16–18, 195
  therapeutic methods in, 20–1, 196–7
  use of assessment tests in, 18–20, 196–7
Eight-step continuum, 10, 132, 134
Electroencephalography, 58

Family (spouses, relatives and significant others), 101–2, 103, 108, 113, 121, 123, 124, 129, 137, 177, 178, 189, 190, 191, 194, 199
Functional analysis, 28, 34
Functional communication, 63, 64, 65, 69, 71
Functional substitution, 33–4

Generalization, 3, 4, 10, 12, 74, 108, 201
Gesture (and pantomime), 6, 7, 8, 130, 131, 132, 133, 171, 179
Gnosis, 3, 8
Group treatment, 9, 71, 88, 113–19
  as learning situation, 116–18
  competition, 118
  homogeneous, 113, 115
  social and emotional needs and, 119
  social effectiveness of, 116
  therapist's role in, 118
  with Blissymbolics, 180, 182

Haptic (tactile) tests, 45, 55–6, 58
Hemi-field viewing (*see* tachistoscopic viewing)
Hemispheric preference, 58
Hemispheric shift (*see* lateral shift)
Hemispheric specialization retraining, 42–59

Immediate constituents, 72
Intelligence, 8
Intensive therapy, 22, 23, 63, 119, 124
Interdisciplinary contribution to aphasia therapy, 2
Interhemispheric transfer of information, 57–8

Language,
  in apes, 29, 71
  propositional vs nonpropositional, 4–5
  second-language learning, 5, 66
  species-specific, 29
Language Master, 175–6
LARSP, 12
Lateral preferences, 44, 55–6, 57, 58
Lateral (hemispheric, dominance) shift in aphasia, 37, 42, 142, 175
Learned helplessness, 40
Learning theory, 116–17
Left hemispherectomy, 43
Levels of representation, 33
Lightwriter, 175–6
Linguistics, 11, 60, 61–75, 63–5
  applied, 5
  approaches to therapy, 61–75
  case grammar, 62
  comparative, 61
  competence and performance in, 4–5
  LARSP, 12
  levels of analysis in, 63–5
  neurolinguistics, 4, 28, 31
  paradigmatic (selection) vs syntagmatic (combination) relations in, 4–5, 67–8
  paralinguistic, 6
  perspective in aphasia therapy, 3, 4–6, 12
  phonology, 8

pragmatics, 63, 64, 69
psycholinguistics, 9, 12, 27–8, 64, 75
similarity vs contiguity, 4
structural, 61, 63
structural semantics, 62
synchronic, 61
syntax, 8, 12
Linguistic perspective in aphasia therapy, 3, 4–6, 12
Lip-reading, 198
Localization of function, 27, 28, 29–31
Logogen system in naming, 87
Loss of identity in aphasia, 91–5

Makaton Vocabulary, 130, 131
Mind-body question, 40–1
Mnesis, 3
Models of recovery of function, 32–5
    collateral sprouting, 33
    compensation, 34
    diaschisis, 32
    functional substitution, 33–4
    levels of representation, 33
    multiple control, 33
    neural regeneration, 33
    neural reorganization, 7
    plasticity, 34
    redundancy of brain tissue, 33
    re-establishment, 7
    relatively ineffective synapses, 33
MRC Psycholinguistic Database, 196, 197

Naming, 76, 85, 116
    effects of word frequency on, 77–8
    episodic memory in, 87
    logogen model in, 87
    phonemic cueing as facilitator for, 6, 76, 82–5, 201
    picture-naming database in, 196, 197
    therapy for, 8, 68–9, 76–87
Naturalistic approaches, 4, 9, 12, 32, 88, 197
Neural inhibition, 7, 59
Neural regeneration, 33
Neural reorganization, 7
Neuropsychological perspective in aphasia therapy, 3, 4, 7–8, 12
Neuropsychology, 11, 12, 25, 61
    and aphasia therapy, 31–8
    holistic school of, 28, 31
Nonverbal cognitive functions, 8, 30, 43
Nonverbal communication as compensation, 11
Nonverbal perspective in aphasia therapy, 3, 4, 6–7, 12

Ongoing evaluation perspective in aphasia therapy, 4, 11–12, 41

PACE, 7
Pantomime (see gesture)
Paraphasia, 63, 125, 138

Personal computers, 175, 176–7
Personal Construct Theory, 90–1
Phonemic cueing 6, 76, 82–5, 201
Phonemic discrimination, 45, 46, 47
Phonological impairment, 135
Phrase structure envelopes, 71–4
Pictographic communication system, 130, 131
Picture-naming database, 196, 197
Plasticity, 34
Psychosocial adjustment to aphasia, 3, 4, 8–9, 10, 12, 19, 88–126, 101–12, 123
    counselling in, 107
    grief process in, 9, 93–4
    interpersonal perception of, 9, 101–12, 194
    perceptual congruence of, 103, 107, 108
    Perceptual Congruence Quotient, 103–5, 112
    perspective, 3, 4, 8–9, 12
Psychosocial perspective in aphasia therapy, 3, 4, 8–9, 12
Psychotherapy in aphasia therapy, 88, 89–100
    good parenting model in, 95–7
    Personal Construct Theory in, 90–1
    reflective questioning in, 99
    techniques of, 98–100
    therapists' needs in 97–8

Qualitively distinct patterns of deficit, 62

Reauditorization technique, 133, 134, 135
Recovery of function (see models of recovery)
Recurrent utterance, 179
Redundancy of tissue, 33
Re-establishment, 7
Regional cerebral bloodflow (rCBF), 38–9, 43, 58
Relatively ineffective synapses, 33
Relatives (see family)
Reorganization, 7
Repetition as facilitator for naming, 76, 78–82
Right hemisphere, role in language, 5, 6–7, 36–7, 42–3, 57–8, 194
Role-play in aphasia therapy, 71

Schizophrenia, 124
Scientific materialism, 40–1
Semantic fields, 68
Semantic impairment, 45, 46
Semiotic system, 6
Senility, 128
Sex and aphasic impairment, 94, 101
Single-case methodology, 16, 35, 38, 53, 58, 193, 194–202
    baseline measurement in, 196–8
    design of, 199–202
    treatment in, 198–9
Significant others in patient's life (see family)
Slow-motion speech, 133, 135
Social regeneration, 114–15
Social skills, 6, 114
Social withdrawal, 114–15

SUBJECT INDEX

Speak and Spell, 175–6
Speech/stroke clubs, 98, 137
Splink, 170, 175, 176, 187–92
Split-brain phenomenon, 30–1, 40, 42
 commissurotomy, 30, 42
 corpus callosum, 30
Spontaneous recovery, 22, 23, 59, 138, 184, 199–201, 202
Spouse (see family)
Subcortical language structures, 39–40
Syntax, therapy for, 69–74
Systematic behavioural perspective in aphasia therapy, 4, 10–11, 12

Tachistoscopic method, 30, 36, 43, 44, 45–7, 55, 56, 57, 58, 186
Telegraphic speech, 36, 134, 183
Temporal lobectomy, 31
Temporal processing in comprehension, 45
Therapy and treatment techniques and methods
 alternative communication methods (see separate heading)
 Amerind (see separate heading)
 articulation drills, 136
 articulograms and articulatory diagrams, 131, 132, 133, 140, 141, 142
 artificial languages (see separate heading)
 Base 10, 10, 11, 47, 48, 50
 behavioural approaches (see behavioural methodology)
 Blissymbolics (see separate heading)
 Brain Function Therapy, 38
 Cloze procedure, 155
 communication aids (see separate heading)
 compensatory strategies, 43
 computer based methods 10 (see also personal computers)
 deblocking method, 5, 41, 67, 85, 163
 eclectic approach to, 4, 127
 eight-step continuum (see separate heading)
 for alexia (see separate heading)
 for agrammatism, 69–74
 for agraphia (see separate heading)
 for apraxia of speech (see separate heading)
 for comprehension impairment, 42–59, 138–145
 for naming impairment (see naming)
 for psychosocial adjustment (see separate heading)
 for sensory aphasia 127, 138–45 (see also comprehension impairment)
 for syntactic impairment, 69–74
 for word-finding difficulty (see naming)
 gestural communication systems, 130, 131, 132, 133
 group treatment (see separate heading)
 hemispheric specialization retraining (see separate heading)
 intensive treatment, 22–3, 63, 119, 124
 learning theory, 116–17
 linguistic approaches (see separate heading)
 lip-reading, 198
 long-term treatment, 22–3
 look-cover-write-check procedure, 154
 Makaton Vocabulary (see separate heading)
 Melodic Intonation Therapy (MIT), 10, 36, 41, 43, 171
 naturalistic approaches, 4, 9, 12, 32, 88, 127
 nonverbal communication as compensation, 11
 PACE, 7
 Personal Construct Theory, 90, 91
 phonemic cueing (see separate heading)
 phrase structure envelopes, 71–4
 preventive method, 36
 proprioceptive neuromuscular facilitation (PNF), 131
 psychotherapy techniques (see separate heading)
 reauditization, 133, 134, 135
 reflective questioning, 99
 repetition (see naming)
 role-play, 71
 self-instructional strategies, 36
 single-case design (see separate heading)
 slow-motion speech, 133, 135
 social skills, 6
 split-sentence technique, 152
 use of video, 71
 visual clueing, 140, 144
 visual communication (VIC), 172–3, 175
Therapist-patient interplay, 41

Visual field preferences (see tachistoscopic viewing)
Volunteers, 9, 15, 18, 21–2, 71, 74, 88, 113, 199
 planning a volunteer scheme, 124–6
 the role of, 121–6

Wada technique, 43
Word-finding difficulty 136 (see also naming)

Author Index

Adams, J.A. 117
Ahearn, M.B. 10, 129
Ajax, E.T. 148
Akhutina, T.V. 64
Albert, M.L. 44, 45, 55, 171
Archibald, Y. 171
Argyle, M. 6, 7
Armstrong, D.M. 40
Aronson, A.E. 128
Artes, R. 101, 102

Bailey, S. 5, 7, 18, 25, 43, 130, 170, 175, 177, 179, 194
Bainton, D. 22
Baker, E. 36, 45, 69, 138, 172
Ball, M. 8
Bannister, D. 90
Barber, J. 68, 85
Barlow, D.H. 53
Barton, M. 43
Basso, A. 17, 23, 41, 138, 139, 171
Bastard, V. 69
Bay, E. 62
Bear, D. 44, 45, 55
Beaumont, J.G. 42
Beauvois, M.F. 157, 158, 168
Bechtereva, N.P. 39
Bennenson, M. 18, 120
Bennett, A.E. 99
Benson, D.F. 37, 146
Benton, A.L. 20
Berman, M. 36
Berndt, R.S. 8, 77
Bernholtz, N.A. 64, 66
Bernstein, J.C. 108
Berry, T. 36, 172
Beukelman, D.R. 101
Beyn, E.S. 36, 67
Bierwisch, M. 5, 62, 67, 69
Binet, A. 27
Bion, W.R. 96
Bisiach, E. 8
Bliss, C. 178
Bloom, L.M. 113, 115, 116
Blumstein, S. 42, 45, 67, 138, 139
Bogen, J.E. 42
Boller, F. 6, 45
Bottorf, L.E. 101
Bowlby, J. 92, 93, 94
Bowling, J.H. 101
Brewer, R.S. 28
Broca, P. 26
Brookshire, R.H. 18
Brown, J.R. 128

Brumfitt, S. 9, 88, 107, 114, 194
Bryant, B. 7
Buck, R. 6, 42
Buckingham, H.W. 8
Buffery, A. 36, 38, 44
Bundzen, P.V. 39
Burton, A. 36, 44
Butler, J. 18, 120
Butler, S.R. 42
Butters, N. 34

Callaway, R. 46
Cameron, H. 192
Cameron, J.A. 130, 131, 132, 172, 173, 177
Capitani, E. 17, 41
Caramazza, A. 8, 64, 77
Casati, G. 138
Castro-Caldas, A. 171
Chassin, G. 69
Chomsky, N. 62, 67
Christensen, A.L. 12, 147
Cicone, C. 7
Clark, E. 18, 179
Clarke, P. 9, 88, 107, 114, 194
Code, C. 8, 9, 11, 12, 25, 30, 37, 38, 42, 45, 88, 93, 130, 175, 194
Cohen, G. 58
Cohen, R. 8
Cole, M. 6
Collins, M.J. 18
Coltheart, M. 11, 12, 14, 16, 38, 43, 150, 193, 196, 197
Cook, M. 102, 108
Cooper, W.E. 42
Crystal, D. 5, 12, 62
Culton, G.L. 23
Cummings, J.L. 37
Czopf, C. 37, 43, 175

Damon, S. 10
Daniels, J.C. 147
Darley, F.L. 15, 17, 20, 21, 35, 38, 128, 136, 137, 200
David, R.M. 9, 12, 14, 19, 22, 193, 194
Davies, C. 66
Davis, G.A. 7, 172, 173
Deal, J.L. 10
Deloche, G. 10, 69
De Renzi, E. 44, 53, 171, 197
Dérouesné, J. 157, 158, 168
De Saussure, F. 63, 67
Diack, H. 147
Dickson, D. 6
Dimond, S.J. 30, 42

Douglass, E. 20
Dubois, J. 62
Duffy, R.J. 6, 42, 93, 101

Eagleson, H. 192
Eaton Griffith, V. 15, 123
Eccles, J.C. 40
Eggert, G.H. 26
Eisenson, J. 143, 145
Elvin, M.D. 69, 70, 165
Enderby, P. 7, 22, 170, 176, 187, 189, 194

Faglioni, P. 17, 44, 171
Farmer A. 31
Fawcus, M. 9, 88, 115
Ferrari, C. 44, 53
Fillmore, C.J. 62
Fletcher, P. 5, 12, 62
Florance, C.L. 10
Flowers, C.R. 101
Fradis, A. 169
Francis, W.N. 77
Fransella, F. 90
Freimann, R. 7, 171
Friden, T. 18
Fust, R.S. 130
Gainotti, C. 7
Galanter, E. 28
Gardener, R.A. 29
Gardener, B.T. 29
Gardner, H. 7, 36, 148, 172, 173, 175
Garman, M. 5, 12, 62
Gazzaniga, M.S. 5, 30, 36, 42, 171, 192
Geschwind, N. 29, 146
Gielewski, E. 5, 25, 127
Glass, A.V. 5, 36, 171, 174, 175, 192
Gleason, J.B. 64, 66, 67
Gloning, K. 63
Godfrey, C.M. 20
Godwin, R. 8, 25, 127
Gogolitsin, Y.L. 39
Golden, C.J. 12
Goldstein, H. 192
Goodglass, H. 6, 11, 18, 28, 31, 43, 44, 45, 58, 62, 64, 66, 67, 69, 76, 77, 138, 147, 171, 197
Goodkin, R. 35
Green, E. 67
Greenbaum, S. 71
Greenberg, F.R. 19
Greenblatt, S. 146
Grewel, F. 62
Grunwell, P. 66

Hagen, C. 16, 17, 22, 23
Halle, M. 61, 62, 67
Hamilton, G. 7, 170, 176, 187, 189, 194
Hargie, O. 6
Harris, A.B. 10
Harris, E.H. 10, 129
Harris, Z.S. 62

Hatfield, F.M. 5, 6, 8, 25, 60, 63, 68, 69, 70, 71, 85, 127, 158, 162, 165, 169, 198
Havighurst, R.J. 114
Head, H. 28
Heard, D.H. 96
Hécaen, H. 62, 146
Hegde, M.N. 74
Heiss, W.D. 63
Helm, N. 66, 171
Helmick, J.W. 101, 102, 108
Hemsley 38
Hermand, N. 69
Heron, J. 97
Hersen, M. 53
Hinde, R.A. 6
Hinshelwood 148
Hjelmslev, L. 67
Hodgins, E. 93
Holland, A.L. 10, 35, 36, 43, 101, 108
Hoops, R. 101, 102
Hopkins, A. 15
Howard, D. 68, 85
Huskins, S. 5, 43, 127, 128, 135
Hyde, M.R. 64, 66, 67

Ingvar, D.H. 38
Irigaray, L. 62

Jackson, H. 5
Jakobson, R. 4, 61, 62, 67
Jenkins, J.J. 62, 128, 129, 133, 137
Jiménez-Pabon, E. 62, 128
Johns, D.F. 8
Johnson, J.P. 43
Jones, C. 68, 85

Kaplan, E. 6, 11, 18, 44, 62, 77, 147, 171, 197
Kean, M.L. 4, 28
Keenan, J.S. 38
Kelley, R.A. 101
Keltor, S. 8
Kelly, G.A. 90, 98
Kenin, M. 23
Kershner, J. 46
Kertesz, A. 18, 23, 35, 192
Kim, Y. 6, 45
Kimura, D, 171
Kinsbourne, M. 43
Kinsella, G. 93, 101
Knudson, A. 192
Koenigsknecht, R.A. 78, 86, 87
Kopp, S. 98
Kotten, A. 64, 169
Kraetschmer, K. 26
Kremin, H. 146, 158
Kubler-Ross, E. 9, 92
Kučera, H. 77
Kurtzke, J.F. 18

Lapointe, L.L. 8, 10, 47, 200

AUTHOR INDEX

Larsen, B. 39, 42, 43
Lashley, K. 28
Lassen, N.A. 38, 39, 42, 43
Laurence, S. 33
LeDoux, J.E. 42
Lemme, M.L. 10, 129
Lenneberg, E.H. 29
Lesser, R. 4, 10, 11, 62, 66, 68, 77, 86
LeVere, T.E. 34
Levine, H.L. 37
Levita, E. 19, 20, 22, 23
Levy, J. 42
Lezak, M. 12
Liberman, R.P. 117, 118
Lomas, J. 23
Lorber, J. 34
Luria, A.R. 5, 28, 33, 34, 36, 45, 62, 69, 127, 128, 130, 132, 137, 138, 139, 147, 150
Lyons, J. 62

Mack, J.L. 45
MacMahon, M.K.C. 62
Mair, J.M.M. 90
Malone, M. 101
Malone, R. 101, 102
Malyshev, V.M. 39
Marcel, A.J. 159, 160
Marcie, P. 62
Marks, M. 16, 17, 18
Marquardt, T.P. 108
Marshall, J.C. 31, 69, 146, 161
McCabe, P. 35, 192
Meikle, M.S. 9, 17, 18, 20, 88, 113, 120
Mesulam, M.M. 7, 42
Meyerson, R. 28
Miller, G.A. 28
Mills, L. 45
Milner, B. 31
Mollon, P. 96
Moore, W.H. 43, 186
Morton J. 6, 60, 68, 85, 87, 159, 162, 163, 168, 201
Moulard, G. 10
Mulhall, D.J. 12, 18, 101, 102, 108, 120
Müller, D.J. 9, 11, 12, 88, 93, 130, 194
Munro, S. 11
Murrell, G.A. 87

Naeser, M.A. 66
Naydin, V.L. 34, 69
Nebes, R.D. 171
Newcombe, F. 45, 69, 146, 161
Newell, A. 28
Newson, E. 96
Newson, J. 96
Nielsen, J.M. 43
Noll, J.D. 37, 43, 74, 175
Norrsell, U. 42

O' Connell, P.F. 31
Ojemann, G.A. 31, 38, 39

Oldfield, R.G. 44
Oscar-Berman, M. 58
Ostreicher, H.V. 7
Palmer, J.M. 101
Parisi, D. 66
Parkes, C.M. 92
Patterson, K. 6, 60, 68, 87, 157, 158, 159, 160, 163, 169, 201
Patterson, M. 6
Pease Myers, D. 76
Pecora, R. 74
Peelle, L.M. 36
Penfield, W. 28, 29
Perepelkin, P.D. 39
Pettit, J.M. 37, 43, 175
Pierce, J. 18
Pizzamiglio, L. 66
Poole, E. 18
Pöppel, E. 148
Popper, K.R. 40
Porch, B.E. 11, 19, 44, 51, 52, 53
Porfert, A. 58
Powell, G.E. 18, 32, 37, 38, 179
Premack, D. 5, 29, 36, 171, 192
Pribram, K.H. 28
Prins, R.S. 23, 41
Prinz, P.M. 7
Ptacek P. 101
Purell, C. 6, 60, 68, 201
Purser, H.W. 8, 25, 42

Quatember, R. 63
Quirk, R. 71

Rasmussen, T. 37
Raven, J.C. 45, 179
Rehbein, L. 58
Reinvang, I. 19
Richardson, J.T.E. 64, 160
Roberts, L. 28, 29
Rochford, G. 66, 68, 78
Rockey, D. 68
Rogers, C.R. 99
Rollman, G.B. 45
Rosen, J.J. 34
Rosenbek, J.C. 10, 129, 132, 134, 137
Rosner, B.S. 33
Ross, A.J. 185, 186
Ross, E.D. 7, 42
Roussele, M. 10
Rowley, D.T. 5, 7, 25, 36, 43, 130, 170, 194
Rusk, H. 16

Saffran, E.M. 77
Sands, F.S. 19, 35
Sarno, M.T. 9, 17, 19, 20, 22, 23, 35, 101, 108
Saunders, C. 6
Saya, M. 184, 185
Schinsky, L. 130
Schlanger, P. 7, 171, 192

Schnitzer, M.L. 5
Schuell, H. 11, 18, 28, 67, 129, 133, 137, 147, 179
Scotti, G. 171
Searleman, A. 37, 43, 186
Seligman, M.E.P. 40
Seron, X. 10, 69
Shai, A. 43
Shallice, T. 158, 161
Shaw, J. 28
Shaw, R. 128
Shewell, C. 5, 6, 60, 198
Shokhor-Trotskaya, M.K. 36, 67
Silverman, M.G. 19, 35, 192
Simon, T. 27
Simon, H. 28
Skelly, M. 130, 137
Skinhøj, E. 38, 39, 42, 43
Smail, D.J. 98
Smith, A. 20, 21, 23, 37, 43
Smith, R.W. 130
Smylie, C.S. 42
Snodgrass, J.G. 196, 197
Snow, C.E. 23, 41
Soh, K. 39
Sommers, R.K. 43
Sparks, R.W. 10, 36, 43, 171
Sperry, R.W. 30, 40
Spinnler, H. 8, 171
Spoehr, K.T. 150
Spreen, O. 20
Statlender, S. 67
Stein, D.G. 33, 34
Stern, G. 18, 120
Storr, A. 98
Swisher, L. 23

Tallal, P. 45
Tanner, D.C. 93
Taylor, H. 16
Taylor, M.L. 20, 101, 108
Teigen, J. 117, 118
Thomae, R. 46
Thompson, J. 32
Trappl, R. 63
Trim, J. 61, 62, 68
Trower, P. 7
Tsvetkova, L.S. 8, 34, 69

Tupper, A. 18, 120

Vandervart, M. 196, 197
Varney, N.R. 8
Vaughn, G. 192
Veroff, A. 172
Vignolo, L. 8, 17, 21, 22, 23, 35, 41, 138, 197
Vinankaya, E.N. 34, 69
Volpe, B.T. 42
Vrtunski, P.B. 6

Wada, J.A. 37
Wagenaar, E. 23, 41
Walsh, K.W. 12
Walsh, M.J. 37
Wapner, W. 7
Warren, C.E.J. 87
Warrington, E.K. 86
Watamori, T.S. 101
Walker, M. 130
Wechsler, E. 9, 18, 88, 113, 120
Weddell, R. 162
Weidner, W.E. 43, 186
Weigl, E. 5, 62, 67, 69, 85, 86, 169
Weiss, D. 18
Welford, A.T. 118
Wernicke, C. 26
Wertz, R.T. 10, 18, 129
Whitaker, H. 11
Whitaker, H.A. 5, 11, 31, 38
Whitehead, S. 114, 115
Whurr, R. 197
Wiegel-Crump. C. 65, 78, 86, 87
Wilcox, M.J. 7
Williams, J. 128
Williams, M. 66, 68, 78
Wilson, D.H. 42
Winnicott, D.W. 96
Woods, B.T. 148
Woods, R. 10
Wulf, H.H. 93

Yule, W. 38

Zaidel, 31, 42, 43
Zangwill, O.L. 7, 8
Zurif, E.B. 36, 64, 172

DATE DUE

NOV 30 1988